To Steph
& Jim,

THE WISH, THE WAIT, THE WONDER

Love
always!
Penny

THE WISH, THE WAIT, THE WONDER

A BOOK OF WISDOM *for* EXPECTANT PARENTS

GAIL PERRY JOHNSTON

HarperSanFrancisco
A Division of HarperCollins*Publishers*

THE WISH, THE WAIT, THE WONDER: *A Book of Wisdom for Expectant Parents*. Copyright © 1994 by Gail Perry Johnston. All rights reserved. Printed in the United States of America. No part of this book may be used or reproduced in any manner whatsoever without written permission except in the case of brief quotations embodied in critical articles and reviews. For information address HarperCollins Publishers, 10 East 53rd Street, New York, NY 10022.

Library of Congress Cataloging-in-Publication Data

Johnston, Gail Perry
    The wish, the wait, the wonder : a book of wisdom
for expectant parents / Gail Perry Johnston. — 1st ed.
      p.   cm.
    ISBN 0–06–250962–4 (pbk : alk. paper.)
    1. Pregnancy—Quotations, maxims, etc.   I. Title.
PN6084.P73J64   1994
612.6'3—dc20   93-33319
                                 CIP

94 95 96 97 98 ❖ HAD 10 9 8 7 6 5 4 3 2

This edition is printed on acid-free paper
that meets the American National Standards Institute Z39.48 Standard.

CONTENTS

For Bev Perry, who wished
and waited and worried and worked.
Also for the wonder of her grandchildren,
Tucker, Bryce, and those yet to be.

NOTE: *I have compiled this collection for some of the same reasons you will enjoy reading it. Anticipation. Curiosity. A little confusion. And eagerness to know everything a person needs to know for a baby to flourish within.*

As I gathered material from hundreds of sources, I found stories that surprised me, saddened me, made me laugh out loud, or merely answered questions. I chose for this book those which would offer the most information and encouragement possible within the confines of two covers.

This book is organized into five parts. The first, The Wish, explores the very beginnings of pregnancy; for a baby is first of all a wish and a prayer in the minds and hearts of the parents. After conception, the baby is a fast-growing reality, evoking even greater hopes and dreams.

Part 2, The Worry, offers empathy and insight while it looks at the fears, unknowns, and sacrifices of becoming new moms and dads.

The Wait encourages couples to make the most of their second and third trimester months: to relish the surprises (e.g., the quickening), to support each other, and to maintain a sense of humor when the waiting gets tough.

Part 4, The Work, refers to labor. The intent of this section is not to recount another gruesome labor story (you'll hear enough of those), but to help prepare expectant parents for whatever their unique experience may be.

The Wonder, the final and most lyrical part, celebrates the moment of birth, the relief when it's over, the beauty of the baby, and the wonder of it all.

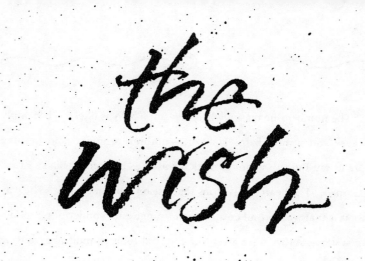

the wish

Not many people can intelligently and comfortably answer the question "Why do you want to have a child?" So, by way of an introduction to the first part, I will briefly present six good reasons to wish for a baby. You will probably identify with one or more of these reasons, and the next time someone asks you the why question (which is likely in these days of population phobia), you will have some real answers. More important, when you experience some of the down sides of pregnancy—the nausea, emotional outbursts, fatigue, weight gain, etc.— you can reassure yourself that you really do know what you are doing, and you really do want a baby.

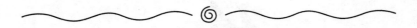

The number one reason why you want a baby is likely to be simply because you want a baby. That's all—nothing profound and nothing more to say. But this is not as weak a reason as it sounds! Blaise Pascal explained, "The heart has reasons that reason does not know." The way I see it is that we were all created with strange and wonderful reproductive systems. As we were given the physical tools to multiply, we were also given the spiritual drive to do so. To be more fulfilled as a woman or a man we just may have to follow those first words spoken to Adam and Eve: "Be fruitful and multiply."

Another reason you want a baby may be because you desire to share your life and pour out your heart into another. Rather than live a life that would be far less complicated, expensive and even painful—should you remain childless—you choose to become a parent because you want to *give*. (Again, there is a spiritual mystery here in that this desire overrides our common sense to choose an easier future for ourselves.) And who would be more needful and hungry for your attention than your very own child?

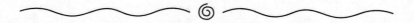

A third reason: you may be looking for a new source of pleasure and meaning. You hope a child will add more enthusiasm, wonder and importance to your life. Although this reason seems a little selfish, it is full of truth! Provided you are an involved, loving parent, a child will certainly enhance your life in a big way. A child is a living gift, given to the parents to enjoy and imposing upon them a role of immeasurable significance.

A similar reason hardly stands alone but is quite admirable. You may choose to raise children to build up your own character, to challenge and stretch everything in you from your patience to your understanding of life. As my friend who has a doctorate in social psychology said, "How can I have empathy for humanity and how can I understand society, which is made up of families, if I have not known for myself the birth and growth of a child and the unconditional, sacrificial love of a parent?"

A fifth motive to have a baby concerns your relationship with your spouse. If you are in love and are fully committed to someone, it is

3

likely that sooner or later you will want to take your love and commitment even deeper. By having a baby, if you are both open and receptive, you will experience a closeness you have not known before as you care for the literal fruit of your love. Caring for your baby and working toward this intimacy, by the way, begins with conception if not before. For the man who has trouble feeling connected to someone yet to be born, caring for the baby may simply mean caring for the woman who holds the baby.

A final reason you may choose parenthood is because you think your child will be someone pretty special—not just for you but for others as well. You hope and expect your child will be a blessing to your own parents, to other loved ones and to the society at large. If such a conviction is combined with love, you can believe quite confidently that the person you raise will contribute more to this world than he or she will take away. As Danny Kaye wisely said, "The greatest natural resource that any country can have is its children."

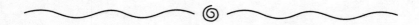

You may have reasons to add to this list. (An "accident" is even a very good one and should be accepted, in time, as something much more.) Whatever your rationale, may you approach your new adventure with boldness. Refuse to entertain any notions that you made a mistake, and may your baby wishes come true!

Remind me never to have kids, I often told my producer whenever we did stories on children . . . children who choose to have tantrums, runny noses, dirty hands and caterpillars. . . . My career, my husband, our home life were fulfilling enough.

Slowly, though, I began noticing pregnant women . . . babies in buggies and Pampers commercials on television. Whatever it was—a biological clock, hormones, or just common sense to want to share one's life—I wanted a child.

JAN YANEHIRO

I never liked babies. I thought they were nonentities. When pregnant, I said that no infant would ever run my life. But then Mark was born. The moment I saw him—that was it. I was awed. I was changed. So much character in such a little body! In the next three years I had three more; each born with distinct personalities and each commanding my deepest devotion. Babies—it was hard to stop having them!

BEVERLY PERRY

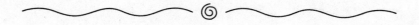

THERE IS NO DESIRE SO DEEP
AS THE SIMPLE DESIRE FOR

companionship

GRAHAM GREENE

During my pregnancy, people told me I wouldn't be able to imagine what motherhood was like—holding my child, being with my child. And now I agree. It's quite different from anything I would have imagined. It is frightening because of the responsibility and also because of the baby's dependence. But it is also the most exciting moment-by-moment thing that has ever happened in my life!

KATHLEEN TURNER

I believe that motherhood is the greatest role of my life. Nothing, not even winning an Oscar, can compete with the pleasure and sense of accomplishment it has given me. I believe that all women feel an instinctive urge to make a family. Some women may use this desire creatively in their work or by living lives devoted to ideas. For me, nothing could substitute for motherhood.

SOPHIA LOREN

enry Rackmeyer, you tell us what is important."
"A shaft of sunlight at the end of a dark afternoon, a note in music, and the way the back of a baby's neck smells . . ."

"Correct," said Stuart. "Those are the important things."

E. B. WHITE

Having a child together—building a family together—seemed a natural progression to the union we began on our wedding day. This little person is, among many other things, a representation of our love for and commitment to one another.

TRISH PERRY

WOULD YOU HAVE YOUR SONGS ENDURE?
BUILD ON THE
HUMAN HEART.

ROBERT BROWNING

The family (is) the first essential cell of human society.

POPE JOHN XXII

There is no finer investment for any community
than putting milk in babies.

WINSTON CHURCHILLL

For the past few years I've been sort of creeping up on a 'yes' decision to have children, but I always thought, "Well, first I have to
give up smoking, lose 15 pounds, paint the kitchen, or get further in
my career." Then I remembered something my dentist, of all people,
told me: "There is never a good time to have your teeth capped, have a
baby, or buy a house."

ANONYMOUS WOMAN QUOTED BY ELISABETH BING

Very few things happen at the right time and the rest do not happen at all.

HERODOTUS

The professor of obstetrics at my medical school used to tell us that there was no right time to have a baby because something else always came up in a couple's professional or domestic life. The corollary of this is that there is no wrong time to have a baby either.

DR. MIRIAM STOPPARD

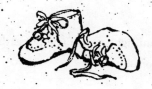

We make up a chart with the days of the month. I set the alarm clock for the same hour every morning, wake up and take Suzanne's temperature, and note it on the chart. Every morning on which we discover a low thermometer reading we make love *immediately* after temperature-taking. One morning we make love *during* temperature-taking. It is, frankly, not the most efficient way to get an accurate reading.

We try to make love every morning during fertile periods, even if we are still asleep, even if we aren't in the mood, even if we have a headache, even if we have had a fight the night before and are still smoldering.

DAN GREENBURG

You will become pregnant right away if you put garlic in the keyhole of your honeymoon suite.

AMERICAN FOLKTALE

You will become pregnant within six months if you lose a pair of earrings.

GUATEMALAN FOLKTALE

You will conceive more easily if you carry mistletoe.

FRENCH FOLKTALE

Immediately after our wonderful weekend of baby-making in Carmel, I started experiencing symptoms. My doctor prematurely gave me a pregnancy test which came out negative. I was upset, but my husband, Steve, was *really* low. Time revealed that I truly *was* pregnant, but the whole experience was very important for me to see just how much my baby meant to Steve. After our second and positive test, we just held each other and cried because we were so happy. Then Steve placed his hand on my stomach and said, "I love you both."

ANDRI WILSON

I always hated the way they planned me,
she took the cardboards out of his shirts as if
pulling the backbone up out of his body and
made a chart of the month and put her
temperature on it, rising and falling, to
know the day to make me—I always
wanted to have been conceived in heat,
in haste, by mistake, in love, in sex,
not on cardboard, the little X on the
rising line that did not fall again.
But then you were pouring the wine red as the
gritty clay of this earth, or the blood,
grainy with tiny clots, that rides us
into this life, and you said you could tell I had
been a child who was wanted. I took the
wine into my mouth like my mother's blood, as I had
ridden down toward the light with my lips
pressed against the sides of that valve in her body, she was
bearing down and then breathing in the mask and then
bearing down, pressing me out into the

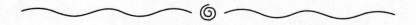

world that was not enough for her without me in it,
not the moon, the sun, the stars . . . not the
earth, the sea, none of it was
enough for her, without me.

SHARON OLDS

We talk of hormonal cycles, ovulation; tell how sperm rush, cells fuse, segment, multiply, travel, embed themselves in the lining of the womb. Yet how did the union of this particular egg and sperm urge life forward to make this child and no other?

The more we learn, greater the wonder, more the mystery.

SHEILA KITZINGER

THE MOST BEAUTIFUL THING
WE CAN EXPERIENCE IS THE

mysterious

IT IS THE SOURCE OF ALL
TRUE ART AND SCIENCE.

ALBERT EINSTEIN

What's miraculous about a spider's web," said Mrs. Arable.
"I don't see why you say a web is a miracle—it's just a web."
"Ever try to spin one?"

E. B. WHITE

I remember a wise teacher of mine saying that the very last area to be conquered in medical science will be the one involving creation itself. It seems as though a higher power is saving this knowledge for itself, knowing full well that it would be too much for a mortal to bear.

DONALD SLOAN, M.D.

As you do not know the path of the wind,
or how the body is formed in a mother's womb,
So you cannot understand the word of God,
The maker of all things.

ECCLESIASTES 11:5, NIV

The mystery of life is not death, but birth; and if there were no economic constraints, I would have an infinite number of children.

ALLEN LENZNER

I was so anxious to conceive that I used a home pregnancy test three months in a row. When I finally saw the "+" on the test, it was like the baby had sent me a little note from somewhere far away—"Yes, I'm here!" I was so wonderfully shocked and afraid to believe his life really had begun.

TRISH PERRY

Much as you may have been prepared for the news, it's always a shock. One student of mine described the confusion she felt when her doctor told her the test was positive. Suddenly she forgot what that meant: was she positively pregnant, or positively not pregnant? For most couples, it truly is an overwhelming moment, and everyone reacts differently to it.

FRITZI KALLOP

Why, when I was told the news,
I felt wings upon my shoes
And gallivanted down the street
Wanting to be indiscreet
And shout to all the world that
I
Was about to multiply.

DOROTHY KEELEY ALDIS

To think that she, Debbie, by offering her body as a temporary
cradle, could influence the pages of family history, could populate
the world with a new citizen, could someday be a grandmother . . .

HELEN GOOD BRENNEMAN

Find Expression

FOR A JOY AND YOU WILL
INTENSIFY ITS ECSTASY.

OSCAR WILDE

I thought for a moment and decided that a man should find out he's going to be a father for the first time in person—not over the phone. The 30-minute drive took me approximately 20 minutes. *I was very excited.*

As I pulled up to the garage where Mike worked, I noticed him and another guy standing by the gas pumps. I walked over to them and stood there grinning. Mike looked up and started grinning, too.

Neither one of us said anything. The other guy kept looking back and forth at us and finally said, "What's going on?"

Mike laughed and said, "She just told me that we're gonna have a baby."

KATHY KUBIACZYK

I'd have to set the stage for Bogie's homecoming that evening—he'd faint when he heard. He didn't faint. I don't know what happened, but after I told him, we had the biggest fight we'd ever had. I was in tears—this moment I'd been hoping for, waiting for, was a disaster. . . . Bogie was full of sound and fury signifying that he hadn't married me to lose me to a child—no child was going to come between us. The next morning he wrote me a long letter apologizing for his behaviour, saying he didn't know what had gotten into him except his fear of losing me . . . but of course he wanted us to have a baby more than anything in the world, he just would have to get used to the idea. He'd spent forty-eight years childless, and had never really considered that being a father would ever become a reality at this point in his life . . .

LAUREN BACALL

Oh, there was a slight sense of horror when Kate first called and said, "Mother, are you sitting down?" I said, "Yes," but of course as soon as she said that, I *knew* what she was going to say. I knew she was pregnant. I knew.

At first there was a sort of denial that this was happening, because how could I possibly be old enough to join that grand generation? Having a grandchild made me look realistically in the mirror and say, "Gee, I'm not as young as I picture myself."

Then, of course, there is this tremendous to-do about what the child is going to call us. Nobody wants to be called Grandma anymore. . . . I have a friend, Gloria, who has been a grandmother for a long time, and she told me, "I didn't want to be called Grandma either, but you know, Pat, in the end you'll fall in line. It's very easy." She said, "The first time I saw that child I threw my arms open to that darling baby and cried, 'Come to your Grandma Glory!'"

PAT MAIN

When the test result was positive, I was shocked. I was so happy and yet so sad that I would never again be alone with my husband. I cried and cried. I felt as if someone had dropped this huge responsibility on top of me and I did not know quite how to begin.

MARY OEI

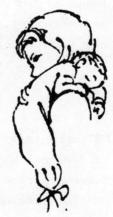

And I sat down on the floor and started to cry. I thought, oh my God, what have I done? We had wanted to have a baby, but wanting to and knowing you are (going to) are two different things. I was crying because, honestly, there was a part of me that said I don't know if I want to love anything again as much as you love a child.

SALLY FIELD

And the truth, I've decided, is that no matter how much you want the baby, there's a good chance that when you get pregnant, your hormones will run so rampant in the early days that you're just miserable and wish you hadn't done it at all. I felt utterly hysterical and miserable at that point, insisting all the while that it had nothing to do with hormones, that I wasn't "emotional" at all (I was irate at the thought). . . . John dared to suggest that pregnant women act a little crazy sometimes. I called him a sexist and a lot of other terrible things, but in secret I think he may be right . . .

DANIELLE STEEL TRAINA

These pregnancy mood swings make the poor, unsuspecting husband think he's walked into an amateur acting class and there's a drama coach yelling to a student: "HAPPY! SAD! ANGRY! HOMICIDAL!" And the student, of course, is his wife.

Barbara would periodically go through all those emotions and more during the course of a ten-minute conversation, so that at times her side of the discussion would sound like: "Oh, honey, I had such a

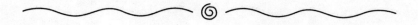

terrible day. My client was so dumb and OH BY THE WAY I HAVE A
BONE TO PICK WITH YOU. WHY THE HELL DO YOU HAVE TO
MAKE THE COFFEE SO STRONG IN THE MORNING? So do you
want to go to a movie tonight? I don't feel so good. I love you."

MARK HALLEN

A curious light has come over Dana these days, as if her pregnancy
wasn't something she carried with her daily, but a new idea
crossing her mind fresh and different each time. She often misses what
I've said in conversation, her cues in the music when she's supposed
to sing.

SARA VOGAN

Three days after the loving act, my stomach felt pumped up with halogen; firecracker cramps were exploding inside of me. I stayed up late that night while my husband slept, giddy with the knowledge that my body was housing another. My cynical self, however, pictured a parasite feeding from me—something foreign was occupying my body. I went to sleep, feeling happy, anxious, and strangely invaded.

According to the fifteenth-century definition, pregnant refers to a state of mind: Ask any pregnant woman about her dreams, her emotional intensity, her wild spurts of energy and the Renaissance definition takes on a timeless quality.

LISA ROCHON

Do I contradict myself? Very well then, I contradict myself. I am large, I contain multitudes."

WALT WHITMAN

We also had discussed our sex life, and Susan was concerned that I would find her unattractive because she was pregnant. In fact, this was never the case. Indeed, I found her more radiant than ever. She never once appeared physically unattractive to me. Emotionally, however, I found that my bond with her became immeasurably stronger. She was now carrying my child, and it became apparent to me that for the first time we were truly bonded together on a common course. Our marriage had been very good up to that point, but in my mind, having a child has turned a very good marriage into an excellent one. In our particular case, Susan always had the stronger sexual drive, but pregnancy seemed to make her more amorous than ever. It seemed that she needed to prove her femininity continually once her body had taken on unusual shapes. I also believe she subconsciously tested my devotion to her during this critical stage of our lives. I hope I passed the test.

RICHARD L. KATZ

Despite the obvious physical connection between the mother and baby before it is born, we must not lose sight of this emotional relationship between the husband and wife throughout pregnancy.

The husband is the single most important influence on his wife. The quality of this emotional relationship is of vital importance to all that is happening.

WILLIAM H. GENNE

No woman is ever so full of love as when she is carrying a child. Whether she planned the circumstance or not, she is . . . carrying love. Man's love, her love, God's love, all joined—united to fashion this precious growing product: life!

Life, the literal fruit of love.

MARJORIE HOLMES

THE DEFINITION OF A *beautiful*

WOMAN IS ONE
WHO LOVES ME.

SLOAN WILSON

Can I regard my pregnancy as anything but one long festival? . . .
I especially remember how at odd hours sleep overwhelmed me
and how I was seized again, as in my infancy, by the need to sleep on
the ground, on the grass, on the sun-warmed hay. A unique and
healthy craving.

COLETTE

A pregnant woman, like a newborn, has very few powers of denial or resistance. . . . At no other time do self-destructive impulses have less a hold on you. Your body will remind you of all the truths you have forgotten. It will tell you, for example, that alcohol troubles your bladder and your sleep; that rich food strains your digestion.

Your memory also rebels at its toxins. Rages and griefs from childhood surface for a while. Then you expel them—as naturally as you stop eating (because you are no longer hungry) or stop smoking (because cigarettes are now physically revolting).

JUDITH THURMAN

In neither the pre- nor post-pregnancy times of my life did food occupy so much of my attention. The focus of my obsession varied from nutritional value to fiber content to blandness (to battle morning sickness) to outright quantity. To a pregnant woman, a single slice of melba toast can, at times, look as appetizing as an ice cream sundae piled high with whipped cream and nuts.

MAUREEN SMITH WILLIAMS

It was frustrating to realize that for the first time in my life, my body was making demands on me that I couldn't override.

I was trying to pursue my career, about which I feel very strongly, and I was forced home for naps. At first I was furious. Later I began to treasure the moments when I was forced to set aside my work for the child within. There's a reality the world should accept. Women shouldn't have to fight to say, "I can do everything at every moment as proficiently as a man." We have to acknowledge that motherhood will take you away from your career, and women shouldn't be penalized for it—just as men shouldn't be penalized for not having wombs.

LYNNE MEADOW

I became spacey during my pregnancy. I was just so focused on my body and its discomforts. Since I was carrying twins, I seemed to move from the first trimester symptoms straight into the third. Along with my rapid growth, however, came a new perspective. The stuff that used to upset me terribly at work was no longer so important.

JOANNE MARQUESE

The worst pregnancy symptom of my first trimester was the nausea and vomiting. Getting sick in itself is an awful experience but to make it worse, I am a visiting nurse so I spend a lot of time on the road. I would be alone on a major highway and would have to pull over to get sick. It was dangerous! The nausea was so unpredictable and nothing would stop it. I had to carry a "survival kit" with a basin and mouthwash wherever I went. It seemed outrageous—to get so sick and then just proceed as if nothing happened! Certain aromas, like greasy foods, seemed to trigger it. Several mornings I visited clients who were frying bacon, and I had to run into their bathrooms. Imagine that—I was sicker than the patients!

ANNE HENNESSEY

By the end of the first month a whole embryo is formed. From head to heel it is a quarter to half an inch long . . . with rudimentary eyes, ears, mouth and a brain that already shows human specialization. There are simple kidneys, a liver, a digestive tract, a primitive umbilical cord, a bloodstream and a heart. The heart is usually beating by the twenty-fifth day. This heart, in proportion to the size of the body, is nine times as large as the adult heart. After a few days of practice it pumps sixty-five times a minute to circulate the newly formed blood . . .

GERALDINE LUX FLANAGAN

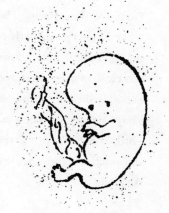

Just a bud
Of a blossom,
And yet—
What a promise
Of beauty
Full-blown
And free

Just a bit
Of a child,
But, oh,
What a vision
Of things
That are
To Be!

PHYLLIS C. MICHAEL

Then I had to deal with the sex of the baby. I didn't want to know, and we had gone through a huge production not to find out. We actually had the doctor's receptionist whiting out all the references in the amniocentesis report so even the doctor wouldn't know. Why should he know if we didn't? But the receptionist forgot to white out the chromosomes. I was flipping through it, and I said, "Oh, my God! That's a Y. We're having a boy."

Ed didn't particularly care, but I had wanted a girl. I expected a girl. . . . I didn't think I knew how to be the mother of a boy: I'm not that close to many men, and I've always been involved in women's issues. I asked my friend Mimi, who has two boys, "How can I have a boy? He's going to be a man!" Mimi said, "Look, you're not having a little boy. You're not having a man. You're having a baby, period, and you'll somehow figure out how to be the mother of that baby. We all do."

JUDY MYERSON

You have a fifty-fifty chance of having a boy or a girl, plain and simple. Incredible as it may seem, there are almost exactly the same number of girls as boys born in the world! When I worked in labor and delivery, we might have nine girls born in a row, but, sure enough, two days later nine boys would bring it to a tie again, and at the end of each year, when we averaged 3,400 deliveries, there would be 1,700 boys and 1,700 girls, give or take one or two.

FRITZI KALLOP

I truly just wanted a healthy baby. However, my husband very much wanted a girl in hopes of naming her after his mother, a wonderful woman who died of cancer. This was so admirable that I found myself hoping for a girl to please my husband. Genetically it is the male's contribution that determines the sex, but I think women tend to feel responsible since they carry the baby.

ANNE HENNESSEY

People ask, "Do you want a boy or a girl?"
The answer is "Yes, of course."

ANONYMOUS

I began to visualize a real child. It was pleasant to imagine the things we might do together: lie under cool shade trees in summer and watch the grass grow; climb mountains and see the world beneath us as the birds see it; read children's stories aloud. It would be a chance to relive the best parts of my own childhood. The delightfully warm sensation of falling in love came over me again.

CHRISTOPHER ORIGER

My dearest . . . I have so many dreams for you. There are so many virtues I would endow you with if I could. First of all, I would make you tough and strong. And how I have labored at that! I have eaten vitamins and minerals . . . gallons of milk, pounds of lettuce, dozens of eggs. . . . I would give you resiliency of body so that all the blows and buffets of this world would leave you still unbeaten. I would have you creative. I would have you a creative scientist. But if the shuffling genes have made of you an artist, that will make me happy too. And even if you have no special talent either artistic or scientific, I would still have you creative no matter what you do. . . . Already I can see how parents long to shield their children from disappointments and defeat. But I also know that I cannot remake life for you. You will suffer. You will have moments of disappointment and defeat. . . . I cannot spare you that. But I hope to help you be such a strong, radiant, self-integrated person that you will take all this in your stride, assimilate it, and rise to conquer . . .

LETTER TO AN UNBORN CHILD, 1941, *BETWEEN OURSELVES*

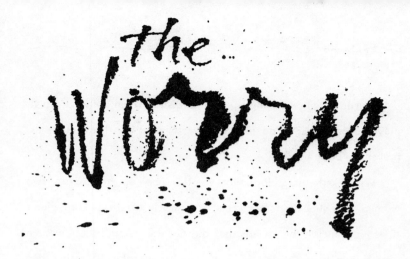

the Worry

Worry is permissible when it motivates us to take care of something necessary and thereby eliminate the worry. If we are concerned about child care, we know that when we find it, our worry will dissipate. But often worry is unmanageable and fruitless, serving only to drain us, dishearten us, and make us very unpleasant to be around.

This kind of worry is softened when we open up to others and ask for reassurance (which is something other than *advice*). When our fears are brought out of the dark corners of our minds and hearts, there is the chance they will wash out in the light and be clearly seen as foolish enemies that need to be discarded.

Worthless worries can also be diminished when we open up in prayer. Especially if we do not know exactly what it is that troubles us, prayer can bring peace.

While gathering information for this book, I came across two women with shocking stories that were nearly identical. Throughout their pregnancies, for reasons they did not understand, these women were extremely opposed to the thought of having baby girls rather than boys. However, they were both carrying girls, and when they gave birth, their emotions went crazy. They were especially troubled when any man, even their husbands, held their newborns. In each case, therapy and prayer revealed the source of their anxieties. They had been sexually abused when very young and feared the same thing would happen to their little girls. Uncovering this dark part of their childhood brought healing. Today they are both very proud mothers, free of their fear and more fulfilled as women.

I hope your fears are not so intense and complicated. I mentioned these women because their stories communicate just how deep the experience of pregnancy can take us. While pregnant, you may struggle with things you have never considered before. Your past, the moral condition of our society, financial matters, even the chemicals in the kitty litter can become a big issue when you're carrying a child.

This section will share with you all kinds of worries during pregnancy. For those worries that can be taken care of, you will be prompted to do so. For those that are merely nagging and hurtful, you will find support, insight, and encouragement from other women and men who have been there.

Pregnancy itself is a healthy, normal occurrence—
humans, unfortunately, are the only species with the
ability to worry about it.

FRITZI KALLOP

We are more often frightened than hurt; and we suffer more
from imagination than from reality.

LUCIUS ANNAEUS SENECA

Pregnancy should be a magical time for a woman, but for me it was
not. I was terrified that I would lose my baby. . . . My emotions
were always at war: yes, I am pregnant and about to become a mother
and soon I will hold my little baby and be the happiest woman on
earth; no, I must not get my hopes up too high or I will invite a
tragedy. I awoke every day relieved to have safely passed another
twelve hours, and went to bed at night with the same thought.

SOPHIA LOREN

There were bad days when I was not quite big enough for the world to know I was pregnant rather than fat. And there were days when I was so tired that I could not move, when my emotional cup ran over, and I thought that I would drown.

There were bad nights too. I had trouble sleeping, and my anxieties grew larger as the hour grew later. I was afraid and I felt guilty for being afraid. I feared the pain, the responsibilities, the way this baby would alter our lives. I feared the unknown. I am no longer a child, I thought in the night. I am the mommy now. I will never again be the child. A little voice deep within me cried, You're not ready. It's diapers and feedings and becoming a haggard housewife from now on, kid. And at two in the morning I believed that voice and cried myself to sleep. I had been such a staunch defender of the positive aspects of having a child that I didn't dare wake Mark and let him see my fear, ambivalence, and weakness.

GINNIE KUHN MITCHELL

I think I have inhibited my feelings because of some silly fear of harming the baby. Of course, tension is more harmful than tears.

CHARLOTTE PAINTER

IT OPENS THE LUNGS, WASHES THE COUNTE-
NANCE, EXERCISES THE EYES, AND SOFTENS DOWN
THE TEMPER.

So cry away!

MR. BUMBLE IN *OLIVER TWIST* BY CHARLES DICKENS

When i can't express
what i really feel
i practice feeling
what i can express
and none of it is equal
i know
but that's why mankind
alone among the mammals
learns to cry.

NIKKI GIOVANNI

I had thought wisdom came with age
that I had learned what I needed
to move on with some grace
if not with ease and dignity
but mid-life years create me child
again.

JUDITH McDANIEL

45

When I became pregnant, I realized that I wanted my mother with me very soon after the delivery to mother, nurture, and care for me. This desire surprised me: I had not needed my mother for years, and suddenly, as I was on the verge of motherhood, my desire for her care and nurturing reemerged.

MYRNA FINN

Blushing, full of confusion, I talked with her
about my
worries and the fear in my body. I fell on her
    breast,
and all over again I became a little girl sobbing
    in her
arms at the terror of life.

GABRIELA MISTRAL

I felt like something was taking over my body, and I was angry about it. I had expected to feel connected to this child in a wonderful, spiritual way. But more and more I had a sense that I was being invaded by this being whose needs always came first and were often in conflict with my own.

I didn't feel like eating at all because of the nausea, but I forced myself to eat well so the fetus would develop properly. I began to be afraid that since my pregnancy was such a disappointment, motherhood would be also. Fortunately, it wasn't, and I adore my child.

SARAH

Of course, everybody knows that the greatest thing about Motherhood is the "Sacrifices," but it is quite a shock to find out that they begin so far ahead of time.

ANITA LOOS

In the dark womb when I began
My mother's life made me a man.
Through all the months of human birth
Her beauty fed my common earth.
I cannot see, nor breathe, nor stir,
But through the death of some of her.

JOHN MASEFIELD

There was another problem as well. Early in my pregnancy my husband told me that I was snoring quite loudly. I was so embarrassed and it only got worse! I finally talked to the doctor and he said many pregnant women snore because the membranes in the nose swell due to the hormonal changes. He said it would probably disappear once I had my baby, but until then, buy your husband earplugs!

KIM NIECE

The output of hormones is colossal. For instance, at any time during an average menstrual cycle, the maximum daily output of one key hormone, progesterone, would be a few milligrams a day; towards the end of pregnancy this rises to as much as 250 mg a day. While progesterone output increases 50–60 times, that of another key hormone, estrogen, increases 20–30 times. . . . No organ escapes the effects of these biochemical alterations.

DR. MIRIAM STOPPARD

Pregnancy is clearly one of the most profound psychological events in a human life. It is the ultimate psychosomatic experience.

DONALD SLOAN, M.D.

My fears revolved around my age. I was not young; the doctor was even younger than me! As my belly grew, I worried about my baby's development, my body's elasticity and my energy level—would I be able to parent a teen when I'm over fifty?

SUSAN JENKINS

SO LONG AS *enthusiasm* LASTS, SO LONG IS YOUTH STILL WITH US.

UNKNOWN

As for the children, I've noticed that there are certain advantages to having older parents, and I'm not sure thay have been suffi- ciently examined or discussed.

In my twenties, I think I was still too much of a child to parent one. . . . But age brings greater self-knowledge and control, ghosts are put to rest, you are less likely to project your longings onto your children, to use them to fill your own needs.

LUCINDA FRANKS

It is wonderful to be young, but it is equally desirable to be mature and rich in experience.

BERNARD BARUCH

I worried about getting fat. I didn't want to tell anyone at my office until I was further along, so I kept wearing my same clothes and letting out the waistbands, hoping they wouldn't notice. This was a mistake because it made me feel there was something "wrong" with being pregnant. I felt much better after I bought real maternity clothes and told everyone that I wasn't just getting fat—I was pregnant! And actually, I rather enjoyed the fact that for the first time in my life, it was okay to put on weight.

MARINA SALUME

To some degree, a pregnant woman must abandon her figure. A trim figure should be your last concern.

SOPHIA LOREN

From here throughout the next seven months, the mother's body begins to change form to accommodate the life inside her. Her bustline falls to her waist, her shoulders and back arch, her knees never speak, and she looks like she has swallowed a thousand camels. There is absolutely NO WAY in the world to look otherwise . . . unless of course, you're on a soap opera. The gestation period of a baby born to a principal on a soap opera is three weeks . . . two if the ratings are in trouble . . .

ERMA BOMBECK

As I continued to grow I decided that dark blue, almost a purple, was one of the more slimming colors for me to wear on the air and I got several maternity outfits in various shades of blue.

One of these outfits was a marvelous knit dress that didn't look like a maternity outfit at all; I wore it often. But the first time I wore that particular dress on the set, David took one look at me and said, "Joan, don't take this wrong, but you remind me of a giant grape." And thus was born the nickname that followed me for the rest of my pregnancy.

JOAN LUNDEN

A body part that receives little attention before pregnancy now becomes a focal point: the navel. As the uterus expands and the skin stretches, the navel is pushed inside out, and under light clothing it's as noticeable as a bull's-eye. One woman I know bandaged the bulge every day. If you have ever wondered what the inside of your belly button looks like, pregnancy is your chance to find out.

MAUREEN SMITH WILLIAMS

S uzanne's belly has not grown as much as she'd expected it would by this time, and she is self-conscious about not showing enough, but her breasts are expanding at an alarming rate. She has gone from a bra size of 34C to 36C to 36D to 36DD to 36DD with a bra extender. It is as if somebody is steadily blowing her breasts full of air like beach-balls. I worry that they will explode.

One day I walk into our bathroom and come face-to-face with Suzanne's latest brassiere. It is enormous. It is draped casually over the shower door. There is something ominous about this brassiere. It is too big. It is somehow . . . unnatural. It has a life of its own. It does not please me to admit this, but I am not comfortable being alone with this brassiere. Watching it carefully for the slightest hint of something malevolent, I back slowly out of the bathroom.

DAN GREENBURG

S tretch marks are trademarks of most pregnancies. They are called striae gravidarum, and I hope knowing their technical name makes you feel better about them. Only rarely does a mother have skin so elastic that it can stretch without them. . . . These marks are most often found on the breasts and lower abdomen and over the hips. They are reddish purple in color, and though the color fades with time, they will not disappear. If you tend to be vain, you will try to make them go away. I suggest that instead of being frustrated, you use this experience to learn a new set of values. Your child will be worth every stretch mark and more.

DR. GRACE KETTERMAN

I worried obsessively about polluting my growing baby's environment. I weakened and had a cup of coffee at a neighborhood gathering and immediately confessed it to my husband, as if he were a priest. He graciously absolved me of any responsibility for our future child's second head or third eye.

TRISH PERRY

Some women metabolize a substance in more harmful ways than others, and the fetus, being more vulnerable, will metabolize it differently still. Caffeine, for example, has a half-life in adults of three-and-a-half hours, but a newborn can take eighty hours to process the caffeine in his mother's breast milk, a premature infant ninety-six hours. Presumably a fetus would take even longer.

WENDA WARDELL MORRONE

Mother and baby have separate blood, but what he receives through the cord is entirely determined by his mother's resources. She takes care of her baby by taking care of herself. . . . However, even if the mother is not eating well during pregnancy, her body will carry reserves if she has been reasonably well nourished before. Also, her biological efficiency is so much stepped up during pregnancy that even mothers who are seriously undernourished have been known to give birth to nine-pound babies.

GERALDINE LUX FLANAGAN

It is a concrete reality that your baby is safer now, deep within the uterus, than it will ever be again! There have been cases of pregnant women who have been in auto accidents or have sustained bad falls, resulting in fractures of the limbs of their unborn babies. Yet those babies healed nicely in the womb without medical help, and were born perfectly healthy!

MARI HANES

One father came to a Lamaze class with a mayonnaise jar and an egg, determined to show everyone just how well-protected the baby really was inside the mother. First, he filled the jar to the top with water and got rid of all the bubbles. Then he cracked the egg, dropped the yolk into the water, and closed the lid tightly. Holding up a crisp, new hundred-dollar bill, he proposed to the class that anyone who could break the yolk without breaking the jar would win the money. Everyone took turns vigorously shaking and tapping the jar—and all the while that little yolk just floated around in a leisurely fashion, without even touching the surface of the glass, let alone breaking. That is kind of what the baby is like, nicely cushioned in the amniotic sac, oblivious to the turmoil of life in the outside world.

FRITZI KALLOP

Although the events leading up to my daughter's being placed in my arms are certainly not the usual pregnancy-labor-and-delivery ones, I went through many feelings and emotional stages, some common to all expectant parents, as I waited for our first child. . . . Sometimes I wondered happy, lazy thoughts—as I weeded my vegetables more vigorously that summer than any summer since—about the baby's sex, size, and looks. I wondered in a worried way about the baby's health, since I had no control over the nutrition, vitamins, toxic substances, or other things affecting this pregnancy. Along with that, I also worried about the birth itself, hoping it would be spontaneous, nontraumatic, and unmedicated. I worried about Apgar scores and about fingers and toes like everyone else does. Things I didn't worry about, things I took for granted and assumed, were that I would love this baby, that she would be my own child, that we would be a family forever.

ABBY JOAN SYLVIACHILD, ADOPTIVE MOTHER

Listen to me, little fetus,
Precious homo incompletus,
As you dream your dreams placental
Don't grow nothing accidental!

ANONYMOUS

We would place our hands on Judith's tummy and pray. Following the growth of our baby as best we could (by reading about the development of embryos in utero), we then asked God to perfectly form the heart, the blood system, the fingers and toes or whatever other parts of the body were being formed. . . . And we prayed also for Judith: we prayed for the days she felt tired—when she felt sick—we prayed for her strength and encouragement—and for a happy day of birth. We were helplessly aware that, beyond a point, there was nothing we could do but wait.

FRANCIS MacNUTT

NEVER UNDERTAKE ANYTHING FOR WHICH YOU
WOULDN'T HAVE THE COURAGE TO ASK THE

BLESSING
OF HEAVEN

G. C. LICHTENBERG

A t some point, by the way, you're going to come up against emotional issues relating to not working, even temporarily. What if a disaster happens while you are gone or—perhaps worse—what if it doesn't? What if the arrangements you have made to cover your job prove to be more efficient than you are? What will you do if your baby still needs you and the job does too? There's no end to the things you can torture yourself with in the middle of the night if you really set your imagination to work.

It's not just a mood swing of pregnancy. For most of us, over the years we have worked, our jobs have become a satisfactory and familiar part of who we are. Thinking of some period of time when we won't have access to that part of ourselves is kind of orphaning.

WENDA WARDELL MORRONE

M any women have two equal fears when they take time off. One is that they're going to hate it; the other is that they're going to like it.

MELANIE KATZMAN, PH.D.

Americans like to believe that combining motherhood and career is guaranteed success under the American Dream—work hard enough and you can do anything. That is not realistic! We must provide the intensive attention children need. They need to have a sense of authority and discipline. They need to be taught how to give and receive love. I have no doubt that if Catherine were small, I couldn't have been the mayor of a big city and still carry out the obligations—and enjoy the pleasures—of motherhood. . . . Be patient with your career and know the special, devoted attention a young child demands will eventually pay off.

DIANNE FEINSTEIN

Sorry, I do not believe that a woman can have it all, at the same time. We might have it all in our lifetime, but we get into a real trap by believing the lie that we can have it all at the same time.

LEE EZELL

Can I let go
of my weekly to-do list
    which I know can be conquered,
    crumpled by Friday
    and my clients who think
    I don't think about babies
    because I'm so happily driven?
Can I let go
if I start to show
    as friends smile stupidly
    as I did for them
    and mother-in-law starts
    sending presents?
Can I let go
of more than I know
    for the love I am told
    is unknown up until
    it is known?

GAIL PERRY JOHNSTON

63

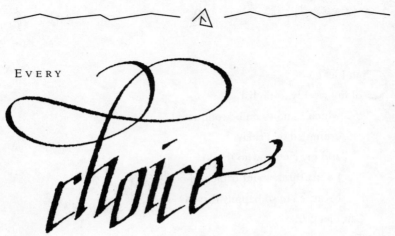

EVERY *choice* IS A LIMITATION.

ELISABETH ELLIOT

From success you get a lot of things, but not that great inside thing that love brings you.

SAM GOLDWYN

I believe that what woman resents is not so much giving herself in pieces as giving herself purposelessly.

ANNE MORROW LINDBERGH

So, the decision was made: I gave up the wardrobe budget, nights out, vacations, worsted wool suits and the frequent flyer program, and quit. I jumped off the ladder of success, checked out of the career world and checked into home. There's no salary that equals the contented feeling I have in my own heart, knowing I've stepped out on a limb and made the right decision.

SUSAN CARROLL AGUREN

And whatsoever you do, do it heartily.

COLOSSIANS 3:23

My husband is seriously anxious about the cost of raising a child today. I resent the horror stories our society has fed us. Most of the calculated costs are just not necessary. So what if our children don't have their own rooms, phones, cars and prepaid college education. We have forgotten that the American dream is about those who have struggled to accomplish great things with little means.

JOYCE TERLMAN

When she reviewed her parenting, she never thought . . . of the good school, the advantages, as they were called. No, what she felt she had given them was her attention: her love, her caring, her willingness to listen.

MARGE PIERCY

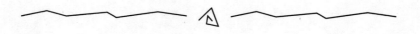

HALF OF THE CONFUSION IN THE WORLD
COMES FROM NOT KNOWING HOW

little we need.

ADMIRAL RICHARD E. BYRD

M any possessions, if they do not make a man better, are at least expected to make his children happier; and this pathetic hope is behind many exertions.

GEORGE SANTAYANA

T here are two ways of being rich. One is to have all you want, the other is to be satisfied with what you have.

UNKNOWN

If my pregnancy was a relatively blissful experience, there were moments of trepidation and sheer panic about introducing a child to the painful insults of reality. One week, after swimming lengths at the pool, I wandered happily into the change room in time to overhear the telling of a tragedy. An attractive blonde woman was describing to a friend how her husband had committed suicide by turning on the car and closing their garage door. I turned away, feeling fiercely protective of the untouched innocence inside me. But my hugely distended stomach also embarrassed me as if I was carrying around too much life for the woman to see.

LISA ROCHON

In the best of times our days are numbered. And so it would be a crime against nature for any generation to take the world's crises so solemnly that it put off enjoying those things for which we were assigned in the first place . . . the opportunity to do good work, to fall in love, to enjoy friends, to hit a ball and to bounce a baby.

ALISTAIR COOKE

I have been wondering what this is going to do to my ambition. I have always been a pathologically ambitious person; it is probably the one quality that defines me most clearly. . . . I'm sure this is a dilemma that new fathers have faced over the ages. But that doesn't make it any less new to me. I will hate myself if I give up any of the professional drive that has always consumed me. But already I feel myself changing. This is going to be very difficult.

BOB GREENE

All changes, even the most longed for, have their melancholy, for what we leave behind us is a part of ourselves; we must die to one life before we can enter into another.

ANATOLE FRANCE

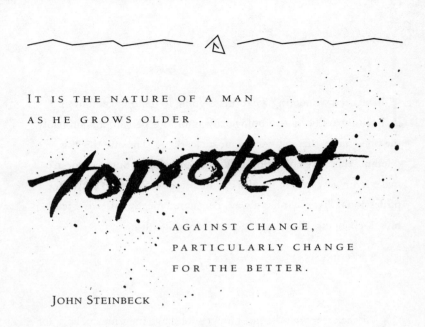

IT IS THE NATURE OF A MAN
AS HE GROWS OLDER . . .

to protest

AGAINST CHANGE,
PARTICULARLY CHANGE
FOR THE BETTER.

JOHN STEINBECK

The night you were born, I ceased being my father's boy and became my son's father. That night I began a new life.

HENRY GREGOR FELSEN

Nothing changes a guy's life more drastically than fatherhood. One day, you're cruising down life's fast lane with the top down, wind in your hair and "Born to Be Wild" blaring on the stereo. The next thing you know, you're poking along near the right shoulder in your station wagon, singing silly songs about some old man who plays knickknack paddywhack on other people's knees. . . . And if you go into this dad thing unprepared, you're bound to end up in a support group for Post-Paternal Stress Syndrome, listening to some tweed-clad simp named Phillip explaining the need for "getting in touch with the inner child."

JIM PARKER

Often the people who are most conflicted about having a baby are those who want no disruption of their established lifestyle. Rather than being delighted with the opportunity to move into a new phase of their own lives, they are afraid that they might be forced to accept an identity that they do not want. . . . Men and women who are eager to experience a "new life" may be those who enjoy the experience the most.

ELISABETH BING AND LIBBY COLEMAN

Life is either a daring adventure, or nothing. Security is mostly a superstition. It does not exist in nature, nor do the children of men as a whole experience it.

HELEN KELLER

Would that life were
like the shadow cast
by a wall or a tree,
but it is like the shadow
of a bird in flight.

THE TALMUD

Don't be afraid to take a big step if one is indicated. You can't cross a chasm in two small jumps.

DAVID LLOYD GEORGE

Perhaps even more important than concerns about finances and physical health are the questions a first-time father has about whether there will be enough love and energy left over for his own needs after the baby is born. Katherine and I really had a good thing going. She had been so loving and nurturing to me . . . that the question of whether she would run out of the positive attention that I was so used to did occur to me. Well, my fears were unfounded: it didn't turn out that way at all. We all love to cuddle in the bed in the early-morning hours when little Alexandra wakes up at the crack of dawn to nurse. . . . Actually I am getting three times as much attention and love than before, and many times this happens before eight o'clock in the morning.

JOHN M. DUSAY

Don't tell me that worry doesn't do any good. I know better. The things I worry about don't happen.

ANONYMOUS

For five and a half months of pregnancy I sneaked around my feelings, demanding no response from my wife or anyone else. I asked other men questions about their pregnancies and got small amounts of information. . . . Mostly, men told me that their pregnancies had gone very smoothly. That was frightening, since I had a great many unsmooth feelings and fears. . . . What was I afraid of? I was afraid that I might not be a good father, that I would not have the patience, the endurance, necessary to make a successful transition to fatherhood. . . . I feared that I would pass out cold in the delivery room and be further emasculated for this great failure. I even feared the deformity of my child. If only I could have heard or read or seen someone else express these concerns, I would have been greatly relieved.

SAM BITTMAN

Even the most unpleasant feelings can fade when shared and responded to. Holding in feelings and needs can lead only to frustration, upset, and alienation. Don't assume your partner knows what you're thinking or wanting. On the other hand, don't assume he or she can't understand your feelings or needs. Parenting begins with conception (if not before), not after your child is born as we've been led to believe. Pregnancy and parenting are two-person experiences. Remember, you are both becoming parents and you need each other. Share your journeys whenever possible and in as many ways as you can.

JACK HEINOWITZ, PH.D.

One's best asset is a sympathetic spouse.

EURIPIDES

It seems incredible that my life is about to change dramatically, and yet I can't really envision how. . . . I hear about "maternal instinct" as though a good fairy flies down to every new mother and sprinkles special maternal dust on her. All I know is that I have not had much luck with house plants I have tended. I hope my performance level with a child is better than with my plants, and that babies are more resilient than coleus.

ROCHELLE BEAL

Hope for the best.
Expect the worst.
Life is a play.
We're unrehearsed.

MEL BROOKS

It is tough. If you just want a wonderful little creature to love, you can get a puppy.

BARBARA WALTERS

Walking down the street I feel immune to any and all harm— and utterly vulnerable. Nothing can touch me yet I am filled with the tenderest life. At home I lie on the bed and watch the show. A foot dances across my belly, an elbow juts. But she isn't causing the sick feeling in the pit of my stomach—that's fear. How will I get through labor? Will I be a good mother? Aren't there some women (not me) who "know" instinctively what to do when a baby cries? What if I can't breastfeed her? What if she hates me? I hate to think of failing this baby in any way.

SUSAN SCHNEIDER

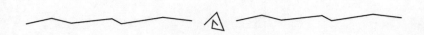

It's a frightening undertaking—becoming a parent. To be totally responsible for the development of a tiny human being is an intimidating proposition. It has been said that the greatest challenge to the human mind is a blank piece of paper. Not so. The greatest challenge is the blank slate of a newborn.

KEVIN KISHBAUGH

A nd you have dreams about your kids. You have dreams that maybe one day your kid will be up there saying, "I'd like to thank the Nobel Academy . . . " Then you have this other dream where your kid is going, "Ya want fries with this?"

ROBIN WILLIAMS

P regnancy is not merely a waiting time. It is a time for working out together what you value in your relationship and what kind of world you both want to create for your child. This is not a question of furnishing a nursery and making things ready for the baby, but of helping each other to change from people who are responsible just for themselves into a mother and a father, with the new responsibility that parenthood brings. A man and a woman need to grow into parents. Then not only a baby, but a new family is born.

SHEILA KITZINGER

Who of us is mature enough for offspring before the offspring themselves arrive? The value of marriage is not that adults produce children but that children produce adults.

PETER DE VRIES

To become a father is not hard,
To be a father is, however.

WILHELM BUSCH

People think responsibility is hard to bear. It's not. I think that sometimes it is the absence of responsibility that is harder to bear. You have a great feeling of impotence.

HENRY KISSINGER

I believe that parents should prepare for the birth of their child by reading everything they can get their hands on and then when the child is born, throw the books away and raise the child by the seat of their pants.

WALTER BRACKELMANNS, M.D.

B ut how do you learn?"
"The way a tennis player learns to play tennis, by making a fool of yourself, by falling on your face, by rushing the net and missing the ball, and finally by practice . . . "

MAY SARTON

We do not want to be beginners but let us be convinced of the fact that we will never be anything else but beginners all our life!

THOMAS MERTON

It's not how far you fall,
but how high you bounce.

ANONYMOUS DAD

There's an old wheeze that says it would be much simpler for everyone involved if second babies could be born first, but since nobody has ever figured out a way to accomplish that objective, we'll just have to go along learning the hard way.

EDMUND N. JOYNER III, M.D.

I come from generations of divorce and alcohol abuse. It's scary but wonderful to have children and an opportunity to do things differently in my own family. Daily, my girls teach me what they need and shed light on what I missed in my difficult childhood. We have a loving home and the history of abuse in my family has been broken.

TERRI MONTGOMERY

The latest research reveals you can best help your baby thrive, not by making sure you take all the "right" steps . . . but by relaxing and being yourself. . . . You don't have to follow all the "right" prescriptions and take all the "right" steps to be a good parent because, frankly, there is no one right prescription or step that works. There are as many wonderful ways to raise a baby as there are babies and parents.

EVELYN B. THOMAN, PH.D.

There's always room for improvement, you know—it's the biggest room in the house.

LOUISE HEATH LEBER, Mother of the Year, 1961

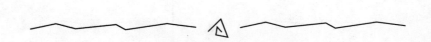

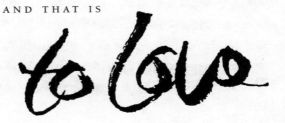

I KNOW OF ONLY ONE DUTY,

AND THAT IS

to love

ALBERT CAMUS

Finally, a footnote. You will never really know what kind of parent you were or if you did it right or wrong. Never. And you will worry about this and them as long as you live. But when your children have children and you watch them do what they do, you will have part of an answer.

ROBERT FULGHUM

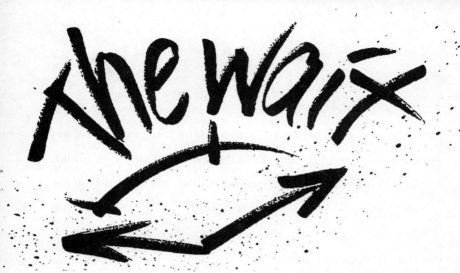

The Wait

We spend so much of our lives waiting. As children we wait to go to school, to grow big. As teens, we wait to drive at sixteen, to be free at eighteen. We then wait and wish for the ideal job, the loving spouse, the affordable house. Ideally, by the time we are having babies, we have developed a little patience and a little confidence in the axiom that "good things happen to those who wait," for inherent in all pregnancies is a nine-month wait.

But, good things can happen *while* we wait as well. Pregnancy can be a time of enjoying your marriage like never before; of making the most of the last months as just the two-of-you. And, if you've been lazy in your efforts to understand each other and build up your marriage, now is the opportunity for a recommitment! Women and men need to "get under each other's skin" at this time and really listen to each other, observe each other, empathize with each other, and make time to discuss views on how a child should be raised. The goal is to become a team by the time the baby arrives, prepared to endure the work of labor and handle the challenges of parenting together.

Pregnancy can also be an opportunity to build relationships with other new parents and to draw closer to those certain relatives and friends who will offer support throughout the years ahead. With all the new experiences involved in becoming moms and dads, you'll want to have good company.

Another way to make good use of the wait is to follow your baby's growth, which is anything but slow. For the baby, things are happening at an amazing speed. For example, on the thirtieth day after conception, the arms are merely rounded knobs, but on the thirty-first day, they become subdivided into hands, arms, and shoulders. The brain on this day is one-fourth larger than it was just two days earlier. In only ten more days, it will have, in miniature, the complex structure of the mature brain. When the baby is ready to be born, one cell has become two hundred million cells, and these cells weigh six billion times more than the fertilized egg!*

One last detail—only 3 to 4 percent of babies are actually born on their due date, so the waiting may persist. When baby is "late," the anticipation, discomfort, and even the phone calls may seem unbearable. I like to think that the purpose of this distress is to make one more and more eager for labor instead of afraid. In any case, this section will speak of such trying as well as tender times during the second and third trimesters. As the German proverb says, "Patience is a bitter plant but it has sweet fruit."

*Geraldine Lux Flanagan, *The First Nine Months of Birth*

This morning I heard my child speak in a heartbeat.
It filled the sterile room, warmed the cold stirrups.
I heard it as a pounding of an elephant herd.
I was filled with its urgency, its unabashed rhyme.

Beat, little tiger, beat on in my ballooned womb.
Let your life song be heard; already you are strong.
Pump furiously, little heartbeat, pump to your own time.
This morning I heard my child speak her first word.

CAROL KORT

I particularly felt, during my second trimester, a sense of well-being
I never experienced before. The nausea had suddenly stopped.
I felt awe and wonder over the changes in my body. I felt very alive,
alert, and completely in sync with my baby—linked spiritually, physically, emotionally.

PATRICIA BARTLETT

Suzanne lies down on an examination table in the sonogram doctor's office, and a female technician moves what looks like a flashlight attached to an electrical cord over Suzanne's belly. The sonogram appears on a video monitor which resembles a very small black-and-white television.

We look in awe at the screen. We have absolutely no idea what we are looking at. The technician points out the fetus's head, buttocks, arms, and legs, and after awhile we can pretty much identify the various parts ourselves.

"There's the head!" I say excitedly.

"Well, uh, no, that's the buttocks," says the technician.

The fetus is in constant motion on the TV screen—turning, wriggling, doing slow somersaults, moving around just the way Suzanne had imagined it was doing in her belly. At one point the fetus scratches its head, as if in embryonic puzzlement. At another it casually crosses its legs at the ankle, as you or I might do while resting them on an ottoman or a coffee table. We are knocked out by our kid's antics.

DAN GREENBURG

The ultrasound was fascinating. As we watched the videotape, I caught a glimpse of my sister and grandmother. I thought I was seeing things but sure enough, my baby is a girl and she looks very much like my sis and my grandmother!

KRISTIN SHOOP

My baby is only inches long and yet it has everything—fingers, toes, even toothbuds! If I'm carrying a boy, he has a penis. If a girl, she is already developing her reproductive eggs. I've been told that real fingerprints exist. This baby, scarcely known to the outside world, is actually carrying the sign of a unique legal identity!

JILL PERRY RABIDEAU

If I could only feel the child! I imagine the moment of its quickening as a sudden awakening of my own being which has never before had life. I want to live with the child, and I am as heavy as a stone.

EVELYN SCOTT

Since my pregnancy was progressing so normally, I expected to experience quickening right on schedule—around the twentieth week. Sure enough, at nineteen and a half weeks, as I sat at my desk at work, Natasha gave me a slight tap. In the days and weeks that followed, these slight taps gradually progressed to stronger kicks, but they were always a delightful experience. Natasha didn't want to play favorites, so at night when I lay beside Dick with my belly against his back, she kicked him too. One night she kicked him so hard that he woke up.

SUSAN KEEL

I felt great during my second trimester. My energy level increased and I started exercise classes (kind of like the dancing hippo scene from *Fantasia*).

The baby's first kick was after one of my exercise classes—I guess he wasn't ready to stop when I was. What a great feeling. I still miss it.

TRISH PERRY

She kicked a lot, more than my son had. I liked it because as long as she was kicking, I knew she was okay. Sometimes I could feel her hiccupping and I liked that too. It made her feel like a real person. Finding out that she was a girl also added to my feeling that she was a real person—not an "it." We called her by name and my husband would put his mouth next to my stomach and say, "When can you come out and play, Jemma?"

MARINA SALUME

Physically, the baby feels like a fish flopping around. First, like a minnow, then a trout, finally a whale.

KIM VALLONE

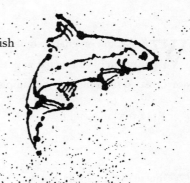

I loved growing bigger! The best feeling was the movement inside. John and I would be in bed reading when all of a sudden my tummy would wiggle like a roller coaster. The movement was *so* profound and exciting that I missed it terribly after our baby was born! Nevertheless, during the pregnancy, the movement kept the three of us very connected.

MEGAN KAHLON

In Kino's head there was a song now, clear and soft, and if he had been able to speak it, he would have called it the Song of the Family.

JOHN STEINBECK, *THE PEARL*

While some pregnant women see only a bulging belly, others are intimately connected with their unborn babies. Such women don't just go swimming, for example, they "take the baby swimming."

ELIZABETH NOBLE

This may sound silly, but we were really getting attached to the little guy. You can only have conversations with something for so long before you start attributing characteristics to it and giving it a personality.

We knew, for instance, that C. M. was up and wanting to be played with every night around eleven. Played with? Sure. We watched Barbara's stomach as it moved, then rubbed where we thought the baby was. Then the baby would move somewhere else, and we'd find it again. Prenatal hide-and-seek, if you will. One night I even tried to play catch with C. M. I rolled a ball over Barb's tummy, and we watched her stomach move after it like an ocean wave.

MARK HALLEN

One of our good friends, Jan Orth, was talking with me and I was sharing with her how children, until they are about three, can often remember being in the womb. So she later asked her son, Matthew (who was then about three), "Do you remember what it was like to be in mummy's tummy?" He started to giggle and the giggle grew into a deep belly laugh: "Oh, sure I remember! I remember I used to tickle you all the time with my foot." Then Jan recalled that when she was carrying him, Matthew's foot would seem to get stuck under her rib cage, causing her discomfort. He'd wiggle his foot, poking and tickling her. So Jan would push the foot back into place; ten minutes later he would have it back under her ribs, poking away. When this all happened, Jan had no idea her baby was playing.

JUDITH MACNUTT

I talked to Robin about the time he swam in my tummy. "The walls were red," he said. Now if you are pregnant, the intense light of a Caribbean island will shine through the wall of your stomach. Children remember things from before they are born. I have a friend who said that his mother played the harp when she was pregnant and now whenever he hears the harp, he immediately fills with happiness. I hope Robin feels the same way about the Talking Heads.

> TINA WEYMOUTH (member of Talking Heads, toured the Caribbean during her pregnancy)

T alking to a fetus is really not as strange as it sounds when you stop to consider that the baby's ears develop by the eighth week of pregnancy and the baby begins to respond to sounds by week seventeen. A number of expectant fathers I interviewed said they talked to their babies in utero all the time, and although they may have felt silly at first, they ended up feeling that it created a real bond between them. It's a good way of overcoming the feelings of exclusion that may make us resent both mother and baby and that may lead us to remove ourselves emotionally from the whole business. And it's just possible that

your unborn baby not only hears you but becomes accustomed to
your voice—hence, in a way knows you even before birth.

DAVID LASKIN

As the baby grew, at almost exactly five months I began having
bouts of breathlessness at night that almost drove me crazy. This
was the single worst thing about this pregnancy. The moment I lay
down I felt as though someone were smothering me. I would attempt
to keep calm for a minute or two, eventually panic and leap out of bed,
taking great gulps of air and feeling incredibly claustrophobic. It was
worse if I ate dinner late (eventually anything after 6 P.M. became
late), or if I ate too much, or if I ate rich foods. A Mexican dinner at 9
P.M. was a near-suicidal event. . . . There were nights when, because of
this, I literally didn't sleep all night. There were nights when getting up
for an hour or two would help, or when sitting up all night would
help. . . . I guess my lungs were just squashed by the baby.

DANIELLE STEEL TRAINA

I was five months pregnant, barely showing, but conscious of every kick and flutter inside my rounding belly. It was all happening so slowly, far too slowly. I felt dragged down, as if the new weight in my body were pulling me under. Some days I felt I could hardly move, and spent hour after hour wrapped in a shawl, dreaming and discontent. I like changes to be immediate and definite, and it seemed then as if all the changes in my life were subtle and organic.

ISABEL HUGGAN

THERE IS NO HEAVIER BURDEN

THAN A GREAT

potential

CHARLIE BROWN

My bladder seemed continually full—I had to urinate frequently—very unusual for me! I would wake up frequently during the night because I had to pee. During the day, I would hope that no one would make me laugh or, worse, hope I wouldn't cough, because that would make me wet my pants. I had little control, and even when I finished peeing, the pressure on my bladder was so great, I couldn't remember if I had just peed or not.

KATHERINE DUSAY

A diagram of your pregnant body from about six months on shows the baby sitting right on top of your bladder. . . . It always amused me how, when visiting those precious little shops along Madison Avenue in Manhattan, if you were not pregnant and asked for the bathroom, the shopkeepers would literally let you die on the floor before conceding they had a bathroom, whereas when you came sailing in with that pregnant belly, they would immediately point you in the direction of the bathroom (the same one that did not exist two years ago) to use "whenever you need it." Take advantage of this temporary gallantry!

FRITZI KALLOP

There definitely is a common experience among most mothers. I can see it in the way that other women looked at my pregnant shape. I used to believe they were thinking, "Oh, I wish that were me," and more recently I was sure they thought, "Am I glad that isn't me!"

It's both.

KATE GRIMES WEINGARTEN

With pregnancy, I discovered how a woman's stomach is suddenly transformed into public property. My stomach, I believed, was swollen with all that is hope and innocence: it was a natural crowd pleaser.

One night, after mentioning absentmindedly that the baby was kicking, three people abandoned a TV thriller to jump from their seats and spread their hands over my stomach. They waited there, looking expectantly at my stomach. The movement had suddenly screeched to a halt. It was as disappointing as a failed fishing expedition. For baby and me, it was the ultimate conspiracy.

LISA ROCHON

There is no such thing as blending into the crowd when you're pregnant. Total strangers come up and ask whether you're going to have "natural" childbirth.

You tell them no, it's going to be unnatural.

Others ask whether you're going to breastfeed the baby.

No, you say. Your husband is going to do it. ("We've always had an egalitarian relationship, and I see no reason to change.")

Still others want to know when the baby is due.

"Baby?" you shriek. "What baby?" (This is especially effective during your ninth month.)

RUTH PENNEBAKER AND LIBBY WILSON

There is one question I hated. . . . It's the pregnant woman's nemesis, the gravida's equivalent of nails being dragged across a blackboard: "How much weight have you gained?"

This question is about as tactful as asking a balding man how much hair he has lost. Think about it: When a woman's stomach swells to the size of a small continent, she's bound to get a little edgy about discussing her weight.

CHRIS KELLY ANDREWS

I bloomed straight out. I stopped traffic. In restaurants hostesses said, "Please don't have your baby in this restaurant." I waited through a very hot August with my ankles swollen beyond all proportion. Swimming saved me—I floated and let the water hold my weight.

DEBBY BOONE

I am a lot less critical of the way my body looked *before* I was pregnant. Maybe I'll be a little nicer to myself *after* this pregnancy!

SUZANNE JOHNSTON

The pattern of weight gain is as important as the total amount. Women generally gain three to five pounds during the first trimester and a little less than a pound a week after that.

If you are in your second or third trimester and already "ahead of schedule" in weight gain, it is important not to cut back drastically in an attempt to reach an "ideal" weight. Your baby will gain most of his weight during the third trimester. Severe caloric restrictions at this stage are likely to shortchange him. It is best to gain about a pound a week until delivery, and to plan on getting back into shape later.

LINDA S. CHIMA, RD

Regardless of weight gain, some pregnancies are all-encompassing and some are not. I'm living proof—I gained the same number of pounds in the same pattern with both my babies, but in my first pregnancy I looked and felt (and moved) like a refrigerator (a side-by-side model), and in the second as though I had tucked a small pumpkin under my dress. The clothes that had barely covered me the first time around hung on me the next time in a sort of war-refugee chic. To your untutored eye, all maternity clothes look alike, but they are not. Some are designed for refrigerator pregnancies and some for pumpkins.

WENDA WARDELL MORRONE

As I got bigger, my center of balance shifted," says Kathy, an exercise instructor. "One day at the supermarket, I reached down for a head of lettuce and fell right into the bin. A shopper had to pull me out by the shoulders. I couldn't right myself!"

MAUREEN SMITH WILLIAMS

Driving downtown for a few bargains, Muriel had attempted to park in a slanting, parallel parking space. It turned out that the space was large enough for her car, but not for her! First, she tried getting out on the driver's side, only to discover that there was not enough room between cars for her clumsy frame. Sliding across the seat, Muriel tried the other side, again to discover that she couldn't get out. After checking to be sure no one she knew had seen her predicament, Muriel looked for another parking place, chuckling to herself as she drove down the street.

HELEN GOOD BRENNEMAN

EVERY SURVIVAL KIT SHOULD INCLUDE A

sense of humor

ANONYMOUS

He who laughs—lasts.

WILFRED PETERSON

Around the sixth month of pregnancy, I began noticing an interesting phenomenon. I'd come home from work and find all kinds of stuff on the floor: paper clips, pens, Barbara's colored markers, mail, cookies, various scraps of paper, and so forth. If I ignored this field of junk, I'd come home the next night to a bumper crop . . .

"Barbara," I said one evening, "how come you're leaving all this junk on the floor?"

"Because," she replied, "when I drop something, I can't bend down to pick it up."

I looked at her and agreed with her plight. Anything at her feet would not only be out of reach, it would be out of sight. I agreed to harvest the floors every night after work.

MARK HALLEN

There is a rule in sailing where the more maneuverable ship should give way to the less maneuverable craft. I think this is sometimes a good rule to follow in human relationships as well.

JOYCE BROTHERS

I liked being pregnant and I enjoyed the special treatment that I received. I did have quite a "nesting" instinct toward the end. I couldn't go into a grocery store and come out without a handful of candy bars. I didn't eat any of them, I just stored them in the kitchen cupboard. Really—it was very strange.

KATHY KUBIACZYK

Gather into yourself
like a bee
the hours that fall open
under the bright shaft of the sun
ripening in heat,
store them
and make of them
    honey days

NUALA NI DHOMHNAILL

For weeks she who had been at best a shiftless seamstress moved around our small cottage in a daze, sorting out pieces of cloth, sewn into garments or raw, sorting and re-sorting them into categories, bundles, neat piles in drawers, in corners, on chairs, for all the world like a nesting mouse. I'd come upon Karen in the bedroom, going through a pile for the nth time; she'd start, look at her hands and recognize what she was doing, and just nod and grin at me in sheepish marvel.

MICHAEL ROSSMAN

She wondered a little
if the neighbors could see
But her baby was sunning,
  her breasts were toughening, turning
  naive white to native brown
And for the first time
  in her eight months of waiting
She was in the present,
  she was floating, falling
  asleep
  like the one
  in her womb.

GAIL PERRY JOHNSTON

Late in the pregnancy you may experience a strange and unsettling moment when you find yourself gazing at your wife with almost total lack of recognition: Could that possibly be the woman I married, that enormously pregnant, waddling, moody, constantly exhausted person who can barely haul herself out of bed, who reads stacks of baby books when she isn't watching the most awful trash on TV, who never wants to go out or have anyone in, whose sole interest is the color scheme of the baby's room, who seems to be in constant communication with her mother? This may be the moment when it dawns on you in a tangible, immediate way that your wife is on the verge of becoming a mother, that she's never going to be "just" your wife anymore. It can make you feel all warm and protective and proud of her, or it can be a little chilling.

DAVID LASKIN

The newness has worn off the thrill of watching your movements ripple across Beth's abdomen. At least two times in the past two days, I've been talking with Beth and she's interrupted suddenly to say, "Watch this baby moving!" And my sudden impulse has been to *feel* interrupted and say, "Hey, Beth, pay attention to me, not the baby." But Beth finds it difficult to listen to anyone else when you are communicating with her through movement.

I think those feelings I have are partially due to my envy of Beth who is able to have such intimate conversations with you. I really am the outsider. Is this how the battle between one parent and a child for the other parent's attention begins? If so, then I am declaring a cease-fire. I don't want to compete with you for Beth's attention; I want to magnify and support her attention for you. But I won't deny my own needs either. So let's agree that we'll each take our turns to both give and receive attention from Beth. All right? All right!

TOM ZINK

My husband disappointed me because I wanted him to mirror my obsessiveness which he didn't. I had an easy pregnancy, but I was still emotional and he would forget to attribute my outbursts to surges of hormones. I am no longer disappointed with him though— he was actually very supportive in his own way. His anticipation came out in the form of "nesting"—he rebuilt the baby's room.

NINA LESOWITZ

During this time it's quite common for couples to make unusual demands on each other as a test of loyalty and devotion. . . . You'll certainly start evaluating each other in the light of your new roles. You may have always had an image of the kind of parent you would want your mate to be, and you'll try to see how he or she measures up to your fantasy. Don't be too hard in your evaluation: remember, you are evaluating yourself in the same way.

DR. MIRIAM STOPPARD

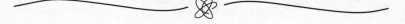

BE NOT ANGRY THAT YOU CANNOT MAKE OTHERS
AS YOU WISH THEM TO BE SINCE YOU CANNOT MAKE
AS YOU
WISH TO BE.

yourself

ANONYMOUS

We had a big fight the night before our baby was born when he said that he was tired of me being pregnant and I said, "Well, how do you think I feel?" That night I slept on the couch! He seemed so cold and unfeeling then, but he was probably just tense and worried, like I was.

MARINA SALUME

So often little things come up
  That leave a pain and sting,
That covered up at once would not
  Amount to anything.

'Tis when we hold them up to view,
  And brood and sulk and fret,
They greater grow before our eyes;
  'Twere better to forget.

ANONYMOUS

I was overwhelmed by the amount of time it takes to make a baby. Nine months seems so long. I was nauseous for the first two months. I spent the third month on my back after almost losing the baby. The middle months I was full of energy at work, but I'd fall asleep at seven. The last months I was just big and thoroughly uncomfortable. Why do women have to go through this agony to have children?

I slowly came to understand as my body worked an embryo into a fetus cell by cell. My thoughts and prayers, hopes and dreams, attitudes and actions evolved. Each day I grew in my heart as the baby grew in my belly. It takes nine months to grow a mother as well as a baby.

KIM VALLONE

When the way is rough, your patience has a chance to grow. So let it grow. . . . For when your patience is finally in full bloom, then you will be ready for anything, strong in character, full and complete.

JAMES 1:3,4, *THE LIVING BIBLE*

My last month of pregnancy was like a final belly dance and I enjoyed a peaceful, symmetrical cohabitation with my guest resident. I understood when the little one would rather go for a walk than have me sit in front of the computer. Gone were the tentative jabs of an earlier time. . . . I followed the undulations with my hand, felt an arm stretch luxuriously or a sturdy leg threaten to kick into my chest cavity.

One midnight, during particularly painful wriggling, I attempted to calm baby with a lullaby. I sang, shyly at first, and then more boldly until the movement stopped and a peace washed through my body. One week before my daughter was born, we were already beginning to understand one another.

LISA ROCHON

I was in such bad shape my last month. I had to stay in bed due to high blood pressure and bleeding hemorrhoids—yuck! But I'll never forget how my husband took care of me. He did all the housework, cooking, and business while I would just lie there. He'd say he was happy *he* wasn't carrying the baby. I was so happy he was carrying me!

PATRICIA BARTLETT

LITTLE BY LITTLE

the time goes by

SHORT IF YOU SING IT,
LONG IF YOU SIGH.

ANONYMOUS

The meeting is imminent.
I am breathless. You crush me.
Breathless too as waiting for a lover
who comes certainly, but at a time unappointed.
My tough little fruit pit, for comfort
will you prefer the womb to the breast?
My skin is taut. You churn in the drum.
Feet kick daringly through the stretched canvas.
I can almost touch the toes
through the bloated belly with its meandering veins.
The meeting is imminent.

You are more real than anyone in my life.
But you are not real.
I carry you everywhere in my gut.
But you are not here.
Soon the fruit blossoms into flower.
The meeting is imminent.

CAROL KORT

Days are so long when we wait. . . . Please stir our minds to remembrance of the beauty of spring after winter, the certain blossoming of the tree, the ripening of the fruit from the seed. Let us know that each day we wait in trust is a part of the process of growing to maturity. Let worry leave our hearts as we learn the technique of waiting with our hands in Thine.

RUTH C. IKERMAN

Nothing great is created suddenly,
any more than a bunch
of grapes or a fig. If you tell me
that you desire a fig, I answer you
that there must be time.
Let it first blossom, then bear fruit,
then ripen.

EPICTETUS

Not since I believed in Santa Claus has time dragged by so slowly as I fantasize about the approaching date and the gift I am going to receive. I keep imagining that warm little body in my arms the way I once visualized over and over again the doll I hoped to see under the Christmas tree. My thoughts are invaded by sweet anticipation!

LUCY BOSWELL

And now, my friends,
All that is true,
All that is noble.
All that is just and pure,
All that is lovable and gracious,
Whatever is excellent and admirable—
Fill all your thoughts with these things.

PHILIPPIANS 4:8, *THE NEW ENGLISH BIBLE*

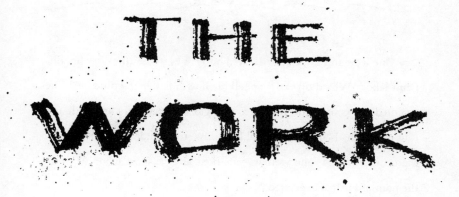

THE WORK

I laughed when I heard how my friend Bob packed a Mary Poppins–type bag for the labor room. Tape recorder, backgammon, granola, thermos, pillows, and so on. I figured he was getting a little carried away with his camping skills. Now I know better. I've read and heard hundreds of labor stories. A couple cannot be too prepared for the possible long hours of labor—of work—ahead. In fact, the entire foundation of childbirth education rests on the concept of preparation. This involves more than packing, of course. It includes learning about the use of medication, the possibility of cesarean birth, and how to work with a birth coach.

One woman I interviewed asked bitterly, even months after her difficult labor, "Why didn't anyone tell me how horrible it would be?" She resented the people and literature that glorified natural childbirth and told me she had "nothing printable" for me to include in this book. On the other extreme, one woman remarked after a short labor, "I think the pain of birth is overrated."

Obviously, no two experiences are alike. (One study claims 25 percent of first-time mothers find labor excruciating, whereas only one in eleven finds it mild.*) The varied stories represented within this part can help you adapt to and accept the unique course of your own labor. Difficult or not-so-difficult, you are approaching possibly the greatest work of your life.

*Dr. Ronald Melzack, *The Challenge of Pain*

I remember sitting in shopping malls during both of my pregnancies, watching all the mothers and children passing by. I kept thinking, "Every one of those kids got here the same way, and their mothers survived. Surely I can do it too." But I never did convince myself. I didn't believe that I could give birth until after I had done it.

SHERRY L. M. JIMENEZ, RN

I couldn't even think about childbirth until the very end of the pregnancy. I was reading about everything else in all the books I'd bought, then skipping the section on delivery. By the ninth month I was still thinking, "I'm not having this baby. I like him right where he is." We were friends. I talked to him. I patted him on what I was sure was the rear end. Many women say, "Get this baby out of me!" I was saying, "You can stay, you can stay."

JUDY MYERSON

I was not looking forward to all this, and the funny thing was that the baby just wasn't real to me yet. They never have been. I have never been able to relate to my children before they were born . . . yet the instant they are born my heart is swallowed by how wonderful they are, how much I love them—but beforehand, zilch. It just seems like a big, ugly bore, and I get so wrapped up in how much it's going to hurt that I'm not real thrilled thinking about the baby. . . . I can't help it. I'm a coward. I was better this time, because my husband was so supportive and wonderful, but I was still mighty scared. I'm not real fond of pain; few people are. I don't handle it that well either (except I do much better than I think I will; most of us do).

DANIELLE STEEL TRAINA

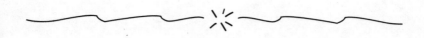

WHAT ONE HAS TO DO
USUALLY

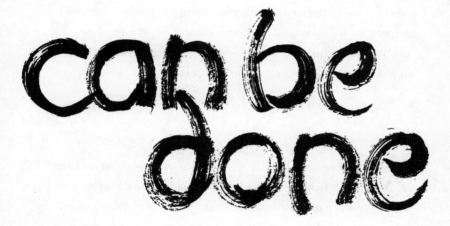

can be
done

ELEANOR ROOSEVELT

Despite all the brouhaha raised by the medical profession over techniques of labor and delivery, by far the most important factors in determining birth outcome are nutrition, prenatal care and preparation (like prepared childbirth classes). . . . It is never possible to eliminate all risk from giving birth or from being alive. But it is up to you, the pregnant woman, to inform yourself.

RAHIMA BALDWIN

A student once said to me, "It never occurred to me not to learn how to give birth. After all, everything I have ever done in my life, from learning to walk, talk, read and write, to preparing myself for a career, I had to learn. It did not come by itself. It seems obvious to me that I had better learn to give birth to my child in order to do it well and as efficiently as possible."

ELISABETH BING, ACCE

When preparing for birth, most families think only in terms of vaginal delivery. But with the national cesarean rate approaching 25 percent, a cesarean birth may become a reality for even the best-prepared parents.

A great deal of controversy rages about whether cesareans are being done too often. However, that doesn't change the fact that many women do have cesareans. It is very important for you to read about and prepare for a possible cesarean, even if you don't think you'll have one. The knowledge you gain will help you to accept, understand, and resolve your cesarean birth experience, should one occur.

ANN CAROL WYMAN, RN

PREPARATION

IS RARELY EASY AND NEVER BEAUTIFUL.

MAYA ANGELOU

Before you can have your baby, you have to attend childbirth classes wherein you openly discuss the sexual organs with people you barely know. You get used to it. You'll get so that when your instructor passes around a life-size plastic replica of the cervix, you'll all hold it up and make admiring comments, as if it were a prize floral arrangement. You'll get to know the uterus so well that you'd recognize one anywhere. Also, you'll see actual color movies of babies being born, so that you'll be prepared for the fact that they come out looking like Mister Potato Head.

DAVE BARRY

Frequent discussions about private matters made those topics seem more ordinary and less sensitive. As commonly as the carpenter calls for a hammer or saw, we in childbirth class used the V-word, the S-word, and the G-spot. I had even become desensitized to the B-word. Baby baby baby . . . I could say it ten times in a row.

SCOTT CRAMER

I had a lot of feelings during prenatal class tonight. Feeling isolated from Beth in her doctor visits, feeling irresponsible that we haven't practiced relaxation and breathing techniques enough, feeling ignorant not knowing what to do in class to support Beth in pushing practice and in labor positions. . . . I decided to share these feelings with Beth on our way home from class. Our talk was very enlightening because of Beth's reassurance that the most important thing is for me to just be there for her.

I've believed for most of my life that I have to be "doing something" to be accepted. Just being there for someone else never has seemed sufficient. . . . "Just be there," she says.

TOM ZINK

Once men are caught up in an event, they cease to be afraid. Only the unknown frightens them.

ANTOINE DE SAINT-EXUPERY

Most of us, on some level, are afraid of labor. If you examine your fear more closely, you'll realize that it's not the pain . . . but the fact that we are not in charge. The fear of lack of control may be worse today because so many first-time parents are older. We've reached a point where we control most of our lives. We're used to it.

WENDA WARDELL MORRONE

To understand the role that control should play in childbirth, imagine yourself in a canoe as it is caught in the rushing waters of river rapids. If you fight the current, using the oars to try to turn the boat, you will end up exhausted without making any progress in controlling the situation. On the other hand, if you give in to the river, letting it wash you along its way, it will force your boat against rocks and fallen branches, adding to the danger as well as the difficulty of your trip. But if you cooperate with the river, letting the current move you forward and using the oars to guide your canoe around the hazards, you will reach your destination in good time. . . . In the same way you use the oar to guide your way around hazards, control should be used to help you through the rough spots of labor, yet your control must be flexible enough to let your laboring body move forward at its own pace.

SHERRY L. M. JIMENEZ, RN

Pain is increased by tension in the body. Keeping any set of muscles contracted for the duration of labor is going to be very uncomfortable. Your uterus relaxes in between contractions, and the rest of your body should be relaxed all the time.

Relaxation is not a passive process. It is a self-directed interaction between your body and mind. How can you stay relaxed during labor? One of your main tools is intention: you are going to sit or lie there, completely relaxed, while strong uterine sensations recur from time to time, and tell your body and your various groups of muscles (especially those in your shoulders and lower belly) to release, relax and stay relaxed.

RAHIMA BALDWIN

A birthing woman's role is to work with her body by relaxing deep within herself and letting her labor happen. Frequently, the loss of energy is more of a problem in labor than the presence of pain.

ELIZABETH NOBLE

Perhaps the single most important technique for easing childbirth is exercise—steady and moderate exercise throughout pregnancy, and exercise and activity immediately before birth. We have come a long way from the constrictive clothing and customs of Victorian life, but we still need a basic change in our way of life if we are to enjoy births without complex backup systems and artificial medications to lighten the load on our out-of-tone bodies.

JUDITH GOLDSMITH

L abour is the natural culmination of pregnancy and simply means hard work.

DR. GRANTLY DICK-READ

F or God hath not given us the spirit of fear;
but of power and of love, and of a sound mind.

II TIMOTHY 1:7

COURAGE— 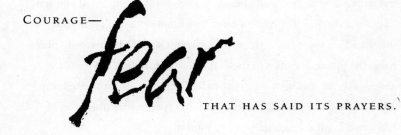 THAT HAS SAID ITS PRAYERS.

DOROTHY BERNARD

Faith is the secret of success: faith in the rightness and beauty of conception and birth; faith in a loving God who made our bodies as they are. Rest on this faith when labor begins, relax all tensions and cares and wait patiently for love's reward.

HELEN WESSEL

Birth is beautifully arranged by nature to bring together the needs of the baby and the capacity of the mother. It is well timed. The baby becomes mature enough to be born just when he is so large that the womb is stretched to its limits. Yet he is still barely small enough to get out through the narrow birth passage. He has no more room to move and no more room to grow. In harmony with the maturity of the baby, the placenta comes to the end of its useful life. This leads to changes in the mother's hormone balance and, in a coordinated way which we do not yet fully understand, the spectacular processes of labor and birth are gradually set in motion.

GERALDINE LUX FLANAGAN

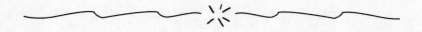

From six months to nine months every day you'll be going,
"Are you OK?"
"I'm fine."
"Are you OK?"
"I'm fine."
"Are you OK?"
"I'm fine."
And you'll know on the ninth day of the ninth month it'll be time
because you'll come home and she'll have the entire house packed in
two small bags . . .

ROBIN WILLIAMS

Everyone tells you how humiliating it would be to go to the hospital if you were only having false labor. And how you would be sent home in disgrace.

This is absolute rubbish.

Should you find yourself in the hospital and realize you aren't really in labor, you have two choices.

One is to apologize profusely to everyone in sight, including the janitor. If you react this way, you will probably be too chagrined to return to the hospital again until your contractions are a minute apart. Then, you will doubtless have your baby in a taxicab, which is considered déclassé.

So by far the better reaction is to show no embarrassment at all. Maintain your dignity at all times. Tell the nurses you were just testing them to see whether they could tell the difference between real and false labor. . . . Announce you just wanted to see the maternity ward and how it was run. Tell them that, on the whole, they did an admirable job, and you'll see them when you feel like it.

RUTH PENNEBAKER AND LIBBY WILSON

My last day of work was Thursday. It was the beginning of the hottest summer in one hundred years. All weekend all I could do is lie on the couch and look totally pathetic.

On Monday morning, my due date, I had a burst of energy. I took the "L" train downtown and stood in line for two hours to get my license renewed. Then walked to Marshall Fields and ate a turkey salad on a croissant in the ice cream shop. I longed for a sundae but didn't dare with the fifty pounds I'd gained. Then, in the lingerie department I tried on thirty gowns before picking that perfect Eileen West robe for the hospital. At the register my water bag broke. My jeans were soaked to the shoes in five seconds with the puddle on the floor growing bigger. As the clerk called for security to escort me to a cab, six little old ladies told me their labor stories.

Of course, I made the cabby's day—"Step on it, Bub!"—that is, until I got out and told him amniotic fluid doesn't sit well in ninety-five degrees!

KIM VALLONE

W hen your water breaks," says Bertha, "it can be only a trickle, or you can lose a quart—nature likes to keep you guessing. But when it happens, a chemical is released which makes you euphoric, so as you're gushing out a quart of water on the carpet in Bloomingdale's Cosmetics Department, you'll have a big smile on your face."

DAN GREENBURG

T he flurry of packing the car distracted me for a while—plus stopping for contractions. I had none of the earlier feelings of dread—just purpose, almost excitement. THIS WAS IT! In the car, Dan said, "Look around, this drive will never be the same again."

JULIE KOVASCKITZ

Walking was what seemed to ease her most. So, through the night we walked, miles and miles up and down corridors and around the birthing room, holding on to one another. When the labor pains became particularly fierce, Perri clutched our shoulders. At intervals, she and Larry breathed in unison as they had practiced. It went on, it seemed to me, endlessly. I tried to encourage her. Soon, I began to wish, soon, for her sake.

SHEILA SOLOMON KLASS

The uterus holds and presses tightly in on the child not yet born, with steadily escalating power. By the end of the first stage of labor it is embracing the baby tightly for one or two minutes at a time. Each hug begins gently and grows tighter and tighter till at the height of the contractions the baby is being gripped fast for 20 to 30 seconds. Then the wave of pressure recedes again and the baby floats once more in its inner sea: it is in labor along with you.

SHEILA KITZINGER

Recent studies on birth memories indicate that some people have total recall of the events surrounding their births. These studies (although for most people these memories are subconscious), provide evidence that your baby's mind is recording her birth. . . . Children between the ages of two and three are often able to recall their births. After three or four, these memories seem to drop permanently from their consciousness. When our little girl, Rachel, was three years old, I asked her if she remembered her birth. She had several memories which indicated some recall. Her first response was: it felt like swimming. When questioned further, she said it also felt like exercise, and she became very tired. She also remembered a bright light.

JUDITH MACNUTT

Soon after returning to bed following my shower, I began to feel the urge to push and the pain was greatly intensified. I told the nurse and she checked but found that I was not yet fully dilated. It was at this stage that I started crying out—something like a primal scream. I was amazed at myself. I would never have believed that I could utter such sounds. For me finding myself screaming was far more embarrassing than exposing myself for all the vaginal examinations and all the other immodest actions and positions required by pregnancy, labor and delivery. The difference, I think, is that it is impossible to be modest and have a baby—I was prepared for that—but I had assumed that one could have a baby without screaming and I intended to do just that. Furthermore, I don't like being out of control, and these sounds were beyond my control. The screams were helpful in that they seemed to release tension. Nevertheless I was embarrassed by them, and each time I let out with one, I apologized profusely to Dick, the nurse and doctor, all of whom assured me I wasn't doing anything wrong.

SUSAN KEEL

With my first baby I felt I had to be brave and not yell or upset anyone. This time I yelled a lot, because I had no painkillers, and it felt great. I heartily recommend yelling instead of these ladylike "Lamaze breathing" exercises as the way to natural childbirth.

MARINA SALUME

Silence is undoubtedly more comfortable to the attendant, but maybe a body needs to release its vocal energy so as to make room for new stamina. What else is a battle cry?

CHARLOTTE PAINTER

Regardless of where the baby is being born, at home or in the hospital, be prepared to leave your sense of embarrassment somewhere else—you will soon realize that what is happening to your wife is the most real thing she's ever experienced. She may groan and moan softly or loudly, become totally uninterested in you, ask you questions you have no answers for ("How much longer?"). So since she's putting her whole self into the labor, it will help her and you if you become as totally involved as possible. You can help her greatly by answering the questions the nurses ask and by making the decisions—she's in no state to think about anything but what is happening to her body—and above all by being positive. Never cast even a shadow of doubt into her mind. Always tell her that she's doing well, because no matter what she is doing, she's doing the best she can. Do not judge her—help her, give her some of your energy. The amount of togetherness you discover during the birth of your child will remain with you and grow for the rest of your lives.

DR. MIRIAM STOPPARD

A lady of forty-seven who has been married twenty-seven years and has six children knows what love really is and once described it for me like this: "Love is what you've been through with somebody."

JAMES THURBER

Father's presence serves two purposes. One is to reduce the anguish of the mother. The other is to increase the anguish of the father. Both seem to me laudable goals. . . . It makes up a bit for the extraordinarily unfair balance of suffering that attends childbirth.

CHARLES KRAUTHAMMER

My husband's involvement, well, I don't know how they would have kept me off the walls without him. I needed him every moment, and he was there for me. He may still have fingernail scars on his back. Strangely, the one time I was distracted (somewhat) from my experience, was when I realized that Hugh was crying—he was hurting for me. It was so touching. I felt, very briefly, like consoling him and telling him it would be all right. Then I felt like a 747 was trying to make a departure from my uterus, and the distraction ended.

TRISH PERRY

WORK IS LOVE MADE

visible

KAHLIL GIBRAN

145

Never before had we, as a couple, reached such complete oneness as we did in helping her make her passage into our waiting arms. It was a long labor, due to her turned position, so we had many hours to spend (from 4 A.M. to 5 P.M.) sharing, working, laughing, praying and finally weeping with great joy when we saw her for the first time. One of the purposes of natural childbirth is to help the parents-to-be work as a team. I marveled at the process of birth, but equally important to me was the oneness with Francis which enabled him to sense and anticipate my fears, pain or loss of control. . . . His presence, holding my hand and praying while I looked into his peaceful eyes, allowed me to draw from him courage and strength to complete the birth. This unspoken level of communication, which can only be communicated by touch and with the eyes, was not attained overnight. It had been worked at and refined since we first met.

JUDITH MACNUTT

If you're a father who is eager to attend the birth of his baby—and most fathers are—you're going to have one of the most amazing experiences of your life and do your wife a world of good. And even if you have serious doubts about attending, odds are it will still be great.

But if you decide you just don't want to be there—or if for some reason you can't be there—don't worry about it. You will have missed one wonderful experience with your child, but the two of you still have millions of wonderful experiences ahead.

DAVID LASKIN

There is this feeling nowadays that if you're not able to participate in the pregnancy and birth, you're doomed. . . . The feeling is that you have to go through this in order to have the best relationship. In two-career couples, people are looking for an executive shortcut to establish a good relationship with their baby. . . . Attending the birth is a wonderful and special thing, but I don't think it means that you bond. It's not enough.

ROB PALKOWITZ

The big trick to being a labor partner is to pace yourself. You may be there for the next twenty hours without a lot of time off. . . . You have to be there for the climax, so don't try to be superhuman. Take time to take care of yourself. If you want to scoot to the cafeteria for a snack, give yourself around ten minutes—long enough to get a sandwich and drink and make a quick stop in the restroom. But don't breathe onions on her when you get back!

BARBARA AND HAROLD HOTELLING

I looked on in wonderment as Jane strained, her face contorted beyond recognition, to release the baby. To avoid being overwhelmed, I concentrated on capturing the power of her effort on film. Right down to the instant of birth the camera shutter framed the event and held back the flood tide of my feelings.

DANIEL J. WISE

The first few hours in the labor room were so easy, they could have been a Lamaze teacher's dream. Every time a contraction would come, Susan would do her breathing, and the pain would pass; it was a breeze. But in the last hours leading up to this moment, the pain had become agonizing. I thought of all the lessons in Lamaze class, from a teacher promising the women that getting through labor would be eminently manageable without drugs; I felt angry, resentful, and helpless as I looked at Susan in the worst pain she had ever experienced. Maybe the breathing exercises were tool enough for some women; but I wished that all of the other expectant mothers in our class could have seen films of something like this, rather than the propaganda of some young mother whizzing her way through labor on a breath and a smile.

BOB GREENE

I felt betrayed somewhat by other women who spared the facts. On the other hand, if I had heard about the pain beforehand I would have been terrified. When you get ready to have a baby, have an epidural and an easy birth. Above all, don't be a martyr about medication-free labor. (I'm sure you have plenty of natural childbirth proponents, so I'm offering the other viewpoint.)

ELLIS

As an intern and as a resident, I had seen lots of deliveries, and I thought I had an appreciation of the pain of contractions. I never anticipated the severity of the pain—it felt like a four-hundred-pound fullback hitting me in the abdomen.

GINNY MAURER, M.D.

The nurse wanted me to sit with the belt on so she could monitor my contractions and the baby's reactions. I was put on a narrow bed, and I couldn't move around. Sitting still through contractions so that you can endure every ounce of pain seems ridiculously cruel to me. I just wanted to move, to let my body be in the position that seemed to help the process along. I wanted to kneel on all fours, or squat, or do anything other than sit still and endure the contractions with a pleasant smile on my face.

I finally lost all desire to cooperate with the nurse and started removing the monitor myself. I told Yogi that I had to have that damn thing off me and to get the nurse in there right away. I'll never forget the way he looked at me: like he suddenly had a mad, totally out of control woman on his hands. I wanted it off and I wanted it off right now. The nurse came in and unhooked me, and I got off the bed and started moving around and squatting. She was really horrified and told me that the floor was dirty. . . . I finally resorted to getting onto the labor bed on all fours and doing cat curls during the contractions.

DIANE BERT

In the middle of everything, I heard people next door saying, "There's Katherine Wentworth in there!" I looked like hell, but I think they thought I should have my hair done and my makeup on!

MORGAN BRITTANY

Jeanie tries to reach down to the baby, as she has many times before, sending waves of love, colour, music, down through her arteries to it, but she finds she can no longer do this. She can no longer feel the baby as a baby, its arms and legs poking, kicking, turning. It has collected itself together, it's a hard sphere, it does not have time right now to listen to her. She's grateful for this because she isn't sure anyway how good the message would be. . . . Something wet and hot flows over her thighs.

"It was just ready to break," the doctor says. "All I had to do was touch it. Four centimeters," she says. . . .

"Only four?" Jeanie says. She feels cheated; they must be wrong. The doctor says her own doctor will be called in time. Jeanie is outraged at them. They have not understood, but it's too late to say this and she slips back into the dark place, which is not hell, which is more like being inside, trying to get out. Out, she says or thinks.

MARGARET ATWOOD

The beginning of labor is a usually joyous social time between our men and ourselves. . . . We breathe together and synchronize our emotions. We share and divide whatever frustrations there might be about the progress of labor or hospital practices. . . . But then as the contractions become more intense, we begin to be less sociable. We spiral down into ourselves, almost hypnotically, to concentrate. Sounds in the room seem far away, time passing has no meaning, suggestions made about our position or breathing seen intrusive. We are deep within ourselves, hoarding strength, almost completely unaware of our men, the babies or the staff. Our total attention is riveted on the irreversible events occurring in our bodies.

DEBORAH INSEL

I can't do this!" Lila screamed.

Every neighbor on the floor above could hear her now for all she cared. Her contractions had been coming two minutes apart for some time, but now something changed. She could no longer tell the difference between one contraction and the next; the pain began to run together in a single line of fire. As each contraction rose to its highest peak, hot liquid poured out between Lila's legs. She couldn't sit, or lie down—she couldn't stand. Ann helped her onto the bed and examined her. By the time she was through, Lila was so wet that the sheets beneath her were soaked.

"Give me something," she begged. "Give me a shot. Put me out. Do anything."

The pain owned her now; it owned the earth and the air and at its center was an inferno. She was in the darkest time before birth, transition, and even though she didn't know its name, Lila knew, all of a sudden, that she could not go back. There was nothing to go back to, there was only this pain—and it was stronger than she was.

ALICE HOFFMAN

I have frequently found that if a trained woman wants to give up in labor, she is either fully dilated or just a few minutes away from it. . . . I say to the fathers or coaches, "Once your partner wants to give up and tells you in no uncertain tones that she has changed her mind about having this baby, or that she'd rather have a caesarean section, or have the baby next year, call the doctor or midwife—you'll find that your wife is either fully dilated or five to ten minutes away from it. The untrained woman wants to give up when she is only 5 cm. or so dilated." Remember it, it's a fairly safe rule.

ELISABETH BING

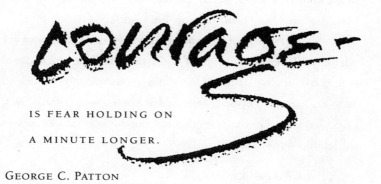

IS FEAR HOLDING ON

A MINUTE LONGER.

GEORGE C. PATTON

The experience in a given moment is never so intense that it cannot be accepted. . . . I knew exactly what my body was doing, and I never pushed as I felt Faith coming down the birth canal. My eyes were wide with amazement and I could feel myself opening—it's such a powerful sensation.

RAHIMA BALDWIN

I was a surfer as a girl and held on to the image of staying on my board. "Keep your balance. Don't fall off!" I chanted to myself. At the same time an old Bob Dylan line wandered through my brain— "And those not busy being born are busy dying."

The extreme pain of labor makes it necessary for many women to ask for painkillers—I didn't but I understand. There are no battle ribbons given for childbirth. For me, though, I wanted to personally grab on to the lifeline so many generations of women have passed down. I can't feel what a medieval mother felt emotionally, but I know what she felt like during labor!

LYNKA ADAMS-KROLL

Is natural childbirth a passing fad?" I find the partisans are as strong as ever, but I notice a discrepancy. They say their fear is reduced, that they do relax and "go with" the labor contractions, but that often at the final stage as the child is born they will accept sedation. . . . Why then? The partisans say that sometimes they are too tired for the final push. It is as if my hunter, with his spear poised upon the pulsing heart of his prey, should decide at that moment to lie down and take a nap.

CHARLOTTE PAINTER

Then they held a mirror down for Julia to see how her perineum was changing, but she only saw a mess of blood, and wanted it wiped away. Now she could see she was flattening out, and the nurse instructed her to place her fingers inside and touch the baby's head! She realized that this little person was close, so very close. She really felt that she was in the hands of God, and God's force was moving through her and this seemed neither bad nor good, just a fact, and even though she thought—"This is agony," the pain almost had an exquisite quality.

LAURA CHESTER

The experience of labor for me was not that bad—it felt one degree worse than very bad menstrual cramps. Even when it was most painful, when contractions were harder and quicker, I felt it was about two degrees worse than cramps. People had scared me—I thought labor was all pain, blood and screams, so I was pleasantly relieved.

BETSY HEBERLING

Eskimo women used to talk about giving birth as being "inconvenient." This is not to say that it was any fun, but they had a remarkably short period of confinement. The women used to sit on their knees while giving birth. If the woman was in a tent or a house when her time came, she would most often dig a hole in the ground and place a box on either side of it to support her arms, and then let the baby drop down into the hole. If she was in an igloo, the baby had to be content with the cold snow for its first resting place. If the birth seemed to take long, the husband would very often place himself behind his wife, thrust his arms around her, and help press the baby out.

PETER FREUCHEN

Day or night, whether or not the bush is dangerous with lions, or with spirits of the dead, Bushman women give birth alone, crouching out in the veld somewhere. A woman will not tell anybody where she is going or ask anybody's help because it is the law of Bushmen never to do so, unless a girl is bearing her first child, in which case her mother may help her, or unless the birth is extremely difficult, in which case a woman may ask the help of her mother or another woman. The young woman was only 50 feet from the werf (the space surrounding a homestead) when she bore her daughter, but no one heard her because it is their law that a woman in labor may clench her teeth, may let her tears come, or bite her hands until blood flows, but she may never cry out to show her agony.

ELIZABETH MARSHALL THOMAS

Courage—a perfect sensibility of the measure of danger, and a mental willingness to endure it.

WILLIAM T. SHERMAN

My mother was, as my doctor put it, a real trouper. She and Dad came to the hospital very early in the morning. Before complications arose, it looked like the baby would come within a few hours after they arrived. Eleven o'clock that night they were still there, despite my protestations. "We're here for the duration, honey," Mom insisted. When we had to go cesarean and I was being wheeled into the operating room on the gurney, suddenly Mom was at my side. "We love you so much, sweetie. You're going to be just fine. We'll be here when you come out, okay, honey?" Tears leaped to my eyes— not from fear or self-pity, but because Mom's affection at that moment meant so very much to me. I was touched in a way I'll never forget.

TRISH PERRY

Transition came without knocking first. And we slipped into the breathing quite naturally. Alice, incidentally, was never so good at breathing as she was during actual labor. Many times during practice she had become discouraged, but somehow, with real contractions, it was easier. She was panting like a Saint Bernard running for a bowl of Friskies.

The most exciting moment came for me at the end of transition, when, with my hand against Alice's back, I felt the baby turn—shoulders, elbows and all. How fantastic to know what it was!

DAVID, QUOTED BY ELISABETH BING

TO A GREAT EXPERIENCE ONE THING IS

ESSENTIAL-

AN EXPERIENCING NATURE.

WALTER BAGEHOT

I was wondering if I could go on like this, thinking I'd ask for some pain medication, when I vomited again. The nurse was nowhere to be found. My husband, Mike, had to clean me up. Then, suddenly, I became convinced I was going to have a bowel movement right in the bed. I was sure of it! Out goes Mike to get me a bedpan and I thought to myself, perhaps we're not having this absolute intimate experience together but thank goodness he's here to help me with all these things! Well, in comes Mike with this nurse who just looks at me and says, "Honey, I doubt it's a bowel movement—it's probably a baby." Next thing I know, a resident examines me and says, "You're ready—PUSH!"

ANNE HENNESSEY

Even after thirteen hours, the baby's heartbeat was strong. I thought to myself, if *he* could still be fighting, I could too. My husband held up one leg and the nurse held the other. I was a horse, soaked in sweat, determined to summon superhuman strength from somewhere for the final push.

JILL PERRY RABIDEAU

And no matter how each particular labor would proceed, it was always interesting to me that all cervixes dilated to ten centimeters—weren't there babies born with bigger or smaller heads than that? I always asked myself this same question and then as I began to be with more couples in delivery, I learned that in fact, miraculously, almost all babies have a biparietal diameter (the widest measurement of the baby's head, at about eye level) of 9.5 to 10.5 centimeters. . . . This measurement was almost absolute. Amazing . . .

FRITZI KALLOP

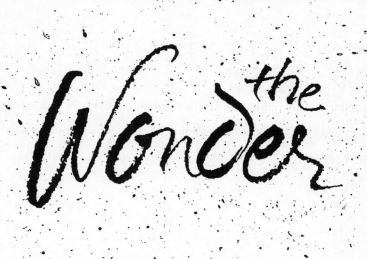

the Wonder

Little needs to be said for this introduction. The fifth section could easily be a captivating book in itself because birth stories are all so extraordinary—full of tension and release, excitement and awe. I've tried to be fair and include words of exhaustion as well as glory, confusion as well as peace, disappointment as well as fulfillment.

I found it curious that one thing was said over and over. Many new parents claimed that their newborn was the most beautiful baby they ever had seen. How could there be so many "most beautiful" babies? An older friend explained, "Years later, when I looked at her pictures, I thought, 'What a funny little creature,' but at the time, she was utterly lovely and I could gaze at her for hours." This is just a part of the wonder celebrated in this last section.

For each ecstatic instant
    We must an anguish pay
In keen and quivering ratio
To the ecstasy

EMILY DICKINSON

There is blood in my eyes. A tunnel. I push into this tunnel, I bite
my lips and push. There is a fire and flesh ripping and no air.
Out of the tunnel! All my blood is spilling out. Push! Push! Push!
It is coming! I feel the slipperiness, the sudden deliverance, the weight
is gone.

ANAÏS NIN

Suddenly everyone seemed to be getting excited. Dr. Chou was putting on his gloves. They just had to get it down under that pubic bone, down and up and out and here. She was becoming more determined now. Down, down, come on baby, the gut crusher of willpower. Every muscle in her neck, face, jaw, shoulders, arms, back and abdomen was straining, pushing, out and under and down. "Just a couple more pushes and you'll have your baby," the nurse's tone brought Julia back again to the bigger reality, that this wasn't just a fight against her own body, but a process that involved another human being, who was working too and being worked. And yet it seemed to go on. Martine held up the mirror, and yes, she thought she could see the littlest part of head crowning, and then a good fifty-cent-size piece of brown wet hair, and that made her push even harder, though she was filling up past the full point, stretching now past all possible limits, burning, and she thought, cool, cool, to no avail, for it felt like a raw hot split. . . . "That's good, Julia," the doctor said. "Just one more push like that one and you've got it." She believed him, and she put all her strength behind it.

LAURA CHESTER

I want my child to come into this world in joy. I have waited for it a long time. . . . And she uttered a single cry, a loud strong one. It did not seem to be a cry of pain, but one of joy. And then her body was pierced by an indescribably sweet, light sensation and she heard the marvelously lusty voice of the newborn child.

LIDIIA NIKOLOEVNA

I pushed for almost an hour. I was holding back just a bit. Then the nice nurse who stayed with me all night pushed my knees to my chest and literally screamed at me "you are going to have this baby now!" All I could see was her face at the end of a long tunnel saying, "PUUUUUUSSSSSHHHHH!" I thought as I bore down, this is as alive as a person gets! My daughter sprung out and stretched as she'd been trying to do for months. She was all vortex cream and red lips. I remembered this later but at the time I passed out!

KIM VALLONE

About midday there were signs that this grandchild of mine was about to emerge, but then nothing much happened and more hours passed. With Perri weaning and unable to bear down with sufficient pressure, the doctor suggested that he might have to help the baby out with forceps.

"No!" Perri said, and she began to bear down with renewed energy.

Suddenly, incredibly, it happened. This plump, round, purplish sack appeared. Tiny arms and legs unfolded and there he was, my grandchild, Benjamin!

"How is he?" Perri asked.

"Perfect," I said, for he was.

For me, this was a transcendent moment. Though I had borne three children, I had never actually seen a child come forth. I was always too busy bearing down, breathing, groaning. . . . That I was there to support Perri and to witness his beginning was a consecration.

SHEILA SOLOMAN KLASS

As Darla's contractions became stronger, she talked more and more about why she was giving up her child and the bond between us seemed as if we were sisters. Finally, I could tell her contractions were so strong that birth was near. I paged the nurse and had barely gotten my greens on when Darla said that she had "to push." We never made it to the delivery room because five minutes later, Darla gave birth to a beautiful boy . . . on the labor bed. When I saw Jayme, I instantly cried and kept saying, "He's so beautiful, Darla." She didn't say anything but was concerned that I was happy he was a boy. She need not have worried. . . . I was ecstatic.

ANONYMOUS WOMAN, coaching the birth of her adopted baby

Ecstasy cannot last, but it can carve a channel for something lasting.

E. M. FORSTER

I was not even fifteen years when I had my first baby. . . . The midwife wouldn't let me lie. She made me walk, my mother on the right and she on the left, and they kept me walkin' and walkin' until my water bag burst, and then they got me up to the bed. From there I couldn't bring that baby, so the midwife she boiled thyme leaf and anise seed and ginger and she gave me that, and that's when the labor start comin' faster and faster. The baby's head crowned, but it was stuck. It was too big. Oh, that pain! The midwife she gave me a washcloth to bite, and I bit right through it. She had to take the baby. She greased her hand with sweet oil, and she caught that baby somewhere by the shoulder, and pulled him out. I passed out.

Oh, but it was worth the while! As soon as that baby was born, oh, the joy! That baby was the beautifullest thing I ever saw. Cecil was so big, thirteen pounds. You look at him, and it seemed he'd been born a long time. His head was right up like he was lookin' at me, looking right into my heart, so I said to the midwife, "Can this baby see?" She said, "No," but I figured he was seeing. I believe that to this day.

PEARL BROASTER

The next time you push you may feel as if you'll explode," Ann said. "You may feel like you're burning."

But Lila had already been a spear of flame; she could dance on red coals now and not feel a thing. She bore down harder, and suddenly the baby's head was free. Lila panted again to stop the urge to push while Ann untangled the umbilical cord from around the neck, and then, with the next push, the entire body slipped out in a rush.

Blood poured from Lila, but she felt strangely renewed. She leaned her elbows on the pillows and lifted herself up so that she could watch as Ann cleaned off the baby and wrapped it in a white towel.

"Is it all right?" she whispered.

"It's perfect," Ann told her. "And it's a girl. . . . " What amazed Lila was how fast it was over, how far outside herself she had gone and how quickly she had returned. Already, the pain she'd felt seemed to belong to someone else.

ALICE HOFFMAN

The pain of birth
  the torture of contraction,
  the panic of transition,
  the abuse of bright lights
  and forceps
Is fast forgotten I am told
  as baby skin is warmed
  by mother's shrunken belly
  and tremors of awe, of love
  overwhelm, overcome
The new woman who is happy
  she, not the man
  gloriously bears the baby.

GAIL PERRY JOHNSTON

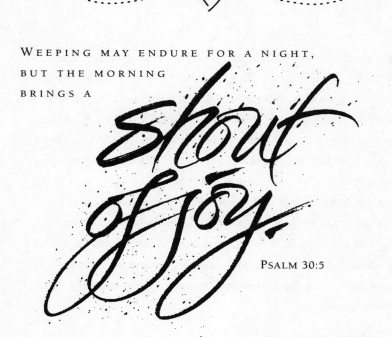

WEEPING MAY ENDURE FOR A NIGHT,
BUT THE MORNING
BRINGS A

shout of joy.

PSALM 30:5

When I first laid eyes on Elizabeth and she on me, it was recognition. I knew her, I knew that was what she looked like, smelled like, sounded like. It was amazing because I could see in her eyes that she knew me too, and was happy to finally "eyeball" me, to touch me. I definitely felt a wave of love flow back and forth.

PATRICIA BARTLETT

I walked back and went to the waiting room, I was scared. I cried. I didn't know what was happening and I felt so locked away from my lover, so helpless. Then suddenly, it seemed too soon, the nurse came in. I think my heart must have stopped at that second. I felt suspended in time. It seemed like a week elapsed before she said, "You have a baby boy," or something to that effect. I think I must have become immobile, because she had to ask me if I wanted to see him. I just can't think of how to describe what happened to me when I first saw him. I had my baby and my wife. At that point the fact that we had him in a hospital or by c-section didn't matter a hoot. With all our thinking and talking about it for months—no, actually for years—there was no way that I could have conceived the absolute joy I felt at that moment.

MARC SCHEVENE

Out of the strain of the Doing,
Into the peace of the Done.

JULIA LOUISE WOODRUFF

Whatever its shortcomings and excesses, though, the return of natural childbirth has been basically good. . . . As a medical student, I delivered 36 babies. Nearly all of them were born to conscious mothers, in the presence of fathers or other helpers. And, as I gazed across the site of what had been such intense pain—at the father, holding the baby I handed him; at the mother, face to face with that baby for the first time—the smiles on their faces said as much as any obstetrics text.

MELVIN KONNER

The instant of birth is exquisite.
  Pain and joy are one at this moment.
Ever after, the dim recollection is
so sweet that we speak to our children
with a gratitude they never understand.

MADELINE TIGER

People say "there's nothing like that first baby." Looking back on
  the births of my sons, I would say both experiences were equally
special, unique. Knowing what I was in for the second time around,
knowing the date of birth, the sex, even the baby's name didn't lessen
the magic and the wonder of it all.

LUCY BOSWELL

I still marvel at the miracle of birth—how every part of my body was made ready for that moment. We have several friends who are obstetricians and midwives who tell us how the harmony of the birth process still impresses them as a miracle. One man we know was an atheist until he witnessed the birth of his first child. He wept openly for the first time in his life when he beheld the miracle of life. You truly become aware of the hand of the Creator when you experience a birth.

JUDITH MACNUTT

Years ago it was unheard of that a woman should wish to see the afterbirth. Today nearly every woman who watches her baby born asks me to show her the placenta. This I do, and point out the bag in which the infant, now lying peacefully in her arms, developed and became a perfect little human being. . . . "Madam, when man can make one of these, he will have reached the foot-stool of the Creator; as I hold this discarded mass in my hand, I am humbled by the limitations of science."

DR. GRANTLY DICK-READ

BEHOLD, CHILDREN ARE A

gift of the Lord,

THE FRUIT OF THE WOMB IS A REWARD.

PSALM 107:43

Perhaps the most vivid account of childbirth that I have heard was given me by Jai Gopal, a little Pardhan boy of about five, who was present at the birth of his younger brother. "What happened?" I asked him. He thought for some time and said, "Fire." He referred to the lighting of a fire to warm the mother, and perhaps to banish evil spirits. "And then?" Another long pause. "Blood!" Another pause. "Water!" Another pause. "Pain. Much pain." Yet another pause. "Life!"

MAIKAL HILLS

After only a few sets of contractions with pushing, the head was delivered. The doctor immediately said, almost shouted, "Sit up and look at your baby!" I will always remember those words and I could actually look down and see her coming into the world. They let me touch her and before I knew it she was on my tummy. This child was amazing—eyes open, already looking at us—and such beautiful, beautiful skin. And such a round head! She was a girl—what immediate joy! I truly felt like the whole world could have ended then and there and I would have been fulfilled. Even now, when I look around at so many people, it's hard for me to believe for each person there was a pregnancy and birth because it is such a monumental event.

ANNE HENNESSEY

At the heart of the universe is a smile, a pulse of joy passed down from the moment of creation. A new parent who holds a baby . . . close against flesh for the first time knows it. And that is the feeling God had when he looked over what he had made and pronounced it good. In the beginning, the very beginning, there was no disappointment. Only joy.

PHILIP YANCEY

When the baby, Kate, was born, she was wrapped in a blanket and put beside me. The first thing she did was to yawn. I was overwhelmed, overwhelmed that she should do such a real thing. Sister Stockman then said, "Now what you need is a good strong cup of tea!" I can even remember that the tea was marvelous. It came in one of those great big canteen cups. It was so strong you could have stood a spoon up in it, and it was very sweet. It was delicious, delicious! It was just what I needed. . . . It's amazing how clearly I can remember. I think it will be just as clear in twenty-five more years.

PAT MAIN

life is only as powerful as its moments.

    a great life is not the result of

    a lot of money . . .

    or smashing success, or prominence.

it is great only in terms of how many

    significant moments there have been. . . .

    i hope i remember the moments.

ANN KIEMEL

S hall I perhaps forget the emotions of this day, my son, in favor of some future minor joy?

You appeared before me, so secure in the support of our doctor's lean hand that it was quite invisible. You alone were there, pale and composed, your flesh undisturbed by the short journey you had just made, even though it was the most important of your life. Yellow moisture clung to the down of your tiny forehead, and yet your brown hair, so surprisingly abundant, curled dry, close against your ears. Your fists were pressed at your chest as if you did not yet know you could open out the fingers. It was the movement of your lips that most impressed me. They curved in a small bow. You seemed to turn your head . . . and as it moved your lips curled upward in discovery, suddenly aware of the feel of some new element. Your tongue made a smack inside, and your lips parted and admitted your first breath of life. You sucked the air inside, and released it with a vocal sound.

CHARLOTTE PAINTER

His eyes widened, then closed tightly, and simultaneously his jaws opened and opened and opened, revealing a space more like the Grand Canyon than a mouth.

I felt him draw a long breath into his lungs, and when he released it in a howl, my mind pictured a cartoon image of pure sound, strong as a hurricane, blowing everything—furniture, hair, trees—in its wake.

MICHAEL DORRIS

The first cry of a newborn baby in Chicago or Zamboango, in Amsterdam or Rangoon, has the same pitch and key, each saying, "I am! I have come through! I belong! I am a member of the Family."

CARL SANDBURG

MY MOTHER GROAN'D,
MY FATHER WEPT,
INTO THE

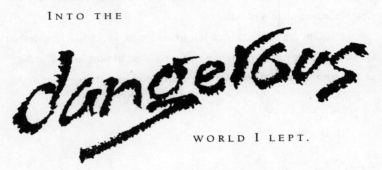

WORLD I LEPT.

WILLIAM BLAKE

I had expected so little, really. I never expect much. I had been told of the ugliness of newborn children, of their red and wrinkled faces, their waxy covering, their emaciated limbs, their hairy cheeks, their piercing cries. All I can say is that mine was beautiful. . . . She was not red nor even wrinkled, but palely soft, each feature delicately reposed in its right place, and she was not bald but adorned with a thick, startling crop of black hair. . . . And her eyes, that seemed to see me and that looked into mine with deep gravity and charm, were a profound blue, the whites white with the gleam of alarming health. When they asked if they could have her back and put her back in her cradle for the night, I handed her over without reluctance, for the delight of holding her was too much for me.

MARGARET DRABBLE

Babies are such a nice way to start people.

DON HEROLD

She sat down and calmly washed the blood from her legs with water from an ostrich eggshell. Then she lay on her side to rest with her baby beside her, and covered the baby from the sun with a corner of her kaross. She put her nipple in the baby's mouth and let her try to nurse. The young woman still said nothing to anyone, but she did open her kaross to show the baby, and one by one we all came by to look at her, and she was not brown, not gold, but pink as a pink rose, and her head was shaped perfectly. At the bottom of her spine was a Mongolian spot, dark and triangular, and her hair, which she shed later, was finely curled and soft as eiderdown.

The father had been away, but he came home a little later and sat stolidly down on the man's side of the fire, his hands on his knee. He pronounced the baby's name softly to himself. Later, when he had no audience, he slipped his finger into the baby's hand. Of course the baby grasped it strongly, and the father smiled.

ELIZABETH MARSHALL THOMAS

Children are poor men's riches.

THOMAS FULLER

They left us alone for a time. We looked at our son. He was so beautiful. I felt a sense of ecstasy. And a love and warmth for Sharon that was thick and palpable and alive. In my head I kept seeing the birth, the body of my son emerging from Sharon's body. I didn't want to lose that image ever. The colors. His crying. Sharon's sounds of joy. We kissed and kissed again and looked at our son. What a woman, what a woman she is, I thought. And she is my wife and she loves me. . . . Maybe the experience has confirmed in both of us our feelings about what a woman is: Not an object. Not a sexual joy, but a sexual partner. Not a frail, fey little thing deserving of sentimental tenderness laced with condescension. But a woman. Brave, enduring, strong, gentle, life-giving and life-enhancing.

GERRY, QUOTED BY ELISABETH BING

As it was in the beginning,
Is now until the end,
Woman draws her life from man
And gives it back again.

NOEL PAUL STOOKEY, *THE WEDDING SON*

frailty,
THY NAME
IS NO LONGER
WOMAN

VICTOR RIESEL

Afterwards—after they laid this gorgeous slimy creature on my belly—I wanted my husband to look into my eyes and say, "Darling, I love you for this." Unfortunately, he is not the sentimental type. My mother understood better and brought me a heart-shaped emerald stone for "a job well done." I think it's very important that women be praised for the birthing process itself: It just might be the biggest achievement of all.

LYNKA ADAMS-KROLL

After our daughter was born, Glenn told everyone I had total control with perfect Lamaze breathing. He must have been in a different room with a different girl. I was drowning in a whirlpool of pain and couldn't even come out of it to scream!

KIM VALLONE

The tiny perfect fingernails and toenails astonished him the most. They were like the small pink shells you scuffed up in the sands of tropical beaches, he whispered, counting them. And, for the twentieth time, he exclaimed, "I don't know how you did it all alone!" His admiration for her bravery sent a glow of happiness through her. It was a new kind of tribute from him. It was a payment in full for all the terrors of her lonely ordeal.

KATHRYN HULME, *ANNIE'S CAPTAIN*

My labor started on Monday night yet I did not deliver until Thursday morning—sixty sleepless hours later. I expected to have a "natural childbirth" yet I ended up with seven tubes coming out of my body. I am entirely sincere when I say that I respect all women who have ever had a baby!

BETSY ZIMMERMAN

The moment of birth. A particle of eternity. And then I experience a marvelous relief from pressure accompanied by a soaring lift of achievement. At the same instant when my flesh is so in contact with actuality, my eyes and heart cannot believe the miracle has happened: one body is now two. A moment later, the next awareness: two bodies becoming one have created a new person. Our handclasp, husband and wife, speaks volumes we cannot say. The fruit of our love is a new human being.

MELISA CASSEL

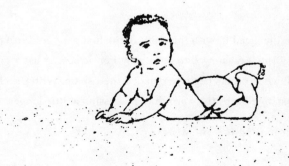

Once the doctor had finished his needlework, I handed our miracle to Dick to hold while I got out of the bed so that it could be cleaned and straightened. Dick took Natasha and held her as though he had been holding newborn infants all his life. That was a delight to behold. I wanted Dick to hold our daughter and to become an intimate part of her infancy, but I admit that I felt a reluctance to let her out of my arms. From the moment of birth I realized that this was the beginning of a long process of watching Natasha grow away from me.

SUSAN KEEL

If one but realized it, with the onset of the first pangs of birth pains, one begins to say farewell to one's baby. For no sooner has it entered the world, when others begin to demand their share. With the child at one's breast, one keeps the warmth of possession a little longer.

PRINCESS GRACE OF MONACO

The skin is the largest sense organ of the body. The sense of touch is actuated early since babies are surrounded and caressed by warm fluid and tissues from the beginning of fetal life. They like closeness, warmth, and tactile comforting. They generally like to be cuddled and will often nestle and mold to your body. The lips and hands have the largest number of touch receptors; this may explain why newborns enjoy sucking their fingers. . . . The sense of touch is a major way that babies comfort themselves, explore their world, and initiate contact.

MARSHALL H. KLAUS, M.D. AND
PHYLLIS H. KLAUS, M. ED., C.S.W.

Taking care of a baby means constant touching. In our culture you're almost never allowed to touch someone except in a sexual context. This is the one time when you can get enough of what you can never get enough of in the whole rest of life—the holding, the kissing, the nuzzling, and the stroking. Not only that, you can get it in public. It's completely sanctioned.

CHRISTINA DAY

When the infant is placed in his mother's arms and at her breast for the first time, appreciate that this is also a new experience for the baby. It is possible that the new baby will immediately take the nipple and nurse vigorously, even right after birth. It is also possible that he will make very little response, and the mother may feel a little worried or disappointed. But remember that the baby has just come from intrauterine life. He has never nursed before.

HELEN WESSEL

Then I called my mother, and I called my best friend, Sandy. "We had the baby! We had the baby!" I gave them each a blow-by-blow description of the birth. I just had to tell the story. I think it's a cathartic thing. It's so intense. So much happens in such a short time that you have to talk about it to make it real. It's how you believe that this baby who has been in your womb, who has been a part of you, becomes a separate person in the world.

There are other reasons why you keep talking about it. Even ninety-year-old women still talk about childbirth. I think you tell the story over and over again to keep from feeling the loss of that experience. To have participated so directly in the creation of life and to have held that life within you is so exciting. . . . And every time you tell that story, you're trying to get back to the miracle.

JUDY MYERSON

I felt sheer relief that my ordeal, and the physical and emotional exhaustion, were over at last. I held her briefly and heard her cry, but my surroundings of bright lights, doctors, and medical equipment, combined with being on my back with feet up in stirrups, were not conducive to fostering initial maternal feelings. I just wanted to be totally by myself. However, as soon as I was being wheeled to my room, I immediately wanted to see my baby and put her to my breast. . . . I am in conflict: I am happy and I am sad; I need to talk and I need to be quiet; I need company and I need privacy; I want to share my infant and I want her all to myself. I am one day into motherhood.

SIMONE BLOOM

Having a baby is like running a marathon. Pregnancy is training; labor the race; delivery the finish line. After the event, exhaustion replaces exhilaration, and aches and pains of all kinds wipe out the "runner's high."

CAROLINE BOVARY

People kept trying to prepare me for how soft and mushy my stomach would be after I gave birth, but I secretly thought, "Not this old buckerina. . . . "

Oh, but my stomach, she is like a waterbed covered with flannel now. When I lie on my side in bed, my stomach lies politely beside me, like a puppy. . . . I'm going to have an awards banquet for my body when this is all over.

ANNE LAMOTT

People talk about the emotions that come when a baby is born: exuberance, relief, giddiness, pure ecstasy. The thought that you have seen a miracle in front of your eyes.

I knew I was supposed to be feeling all of those things, and of course I did. But the dominant emotion inside me was a more basic one. I was scared; scared of what I knew was sure to come, and more scared about what I didn't know. I am of a generation that has made self-indulgence a kind of secular religion. I looked down at that baby, and suddenly I felt that a whole part of my life had just ended, been cut off, and I was beginning something for which I had no preparation.

That's what went through me as I watched my baby enter the world; a sense of fear unlike any I have felt in my life.

BOB GREENE

About a quarter of the men in our university studies found the birth experience rather stressful. Half were intensely fatigued, almost as much as the mother.

RAMONA MERCER, PH.D.

THE THING ABOUT HAVING A BABY
IS THAT
THEREAFTER 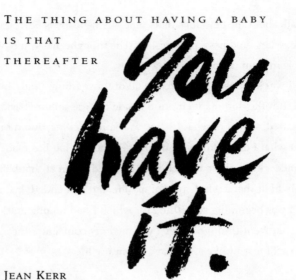 *you have it.*

JEAN KERR

It is a good idea to evaluate what you both felt about the baby's birth so that you can reconcile what you had imagined it would be like and what you actually experienced. . . . For some couples the birth experience is truly fabulous, but for many others it's an experience they are glad to put behind them.

If your baby was delivered by cesarean section, then you may be somewhat more depleted as new parents. . . . You both have many feelings to sort out after the baby is safely delivered, especially because most cesareans are unexpected.

TRACY HOTCHNER

Cesarean sections . . . occur in approximately 20 percent of all births. The Cesarean rate has not always been this high. Fifteen or 20 years ago, when the rate was about five percent, an abdominal delivery was considered a sign of obstetrical failure. Today, unfortunately, many see it as a sign of maternal failure. This attitude places blame on the woman for an event that results from a combination of factors. . . . Realize that no matter what happened, you did your best under difficult circumstances. When someone tells you what a great job you did, believe it and say, "Thanks!" See, hear, smell, and feel how marvelous your baby is. She took nine months of your life and some very hard work to get here, and she hasn't got a single complaint about how you behaved during her birth.

SHERRY L. M. JIMENEZ, RN

M y day of labor was the worst day of my life, but isn't it curious that the worst day of my life produced the best thing in my life?

BETSY DEPEW

I t's easy to become competitive about the amount of anesthesia you had, the number of hours you were in labor, of how strong a feeling of maternal bonding you felt at your first sight of the baby. . . . If the heavens opened up for you at the moment of birth, that's a bonus, but it is also only one experience of a lifetime. It's the accumulation of experiences, some of them unpleasant, that turns us into parents.

WENDA WARDELL MORRONE

I t isn't always love at first sight: Two in ten parents admit it took weeks or even months before they were smitten with their offspring. And two-thirds say newborn babies are "intimidating."

CARIN RUBENSTEIN, PH.D.

A newborn baby is merely a small, noisy object, slightly fuzzy on one end, with no distinguishing marks to speak of except a mouth, and in color either a salmon pink or a deep sorrel, depending on whether it is going to grow up a blonde or a brunette. But to its immediate family, it is without question the most phenomenal, the most astonishing, the most absolutely unparalleled thing that has yet occurred in the entire history of this planet.

IRVIN S. COBB

The first duty owed to the child is to ascertain which parent it resembles. Sometimes it pleases a father to have it said his baby looks like him and sometimes it makes a father want to fight; other times to say a baby looks like its father is base libel on the baby, especially if the baby is pretty and the father is a lantern-jawed, wall-eyed homely old piker.

NEWTON NEWKIRK

My day-old son is plenty scrawny,
His mouth is wide with screams, or yawny,
His ears seem larger than he's needing,
His nose is flat, his chin's receding,
His skin is very, very red,
He has no hair upon his head,
And yet I'm proud as proud can be,
To hear you say he looks like me.

RICHARD ARMOUR

Then she had a girl, Melanie, a little creature so immediately happy with herself that it seemed to Emma she had been created just to make everyone feel better.

LARRY MCMURTRY, *TERMS OF ENDEARMENT*

Of thee I sing, baby,
You have got that certain thing, baby,
Shining star and inspiration
Worthy of a mighty nation,
Of thee I sing!

IRA GERSHWIN

For the old view of a baby as a blank tablet . . . or an infinitely mal-
leable blob of clay has in recent years given way to the recognition that babies are born with specific temperaments and coping
capacities. The growing field of infant research has established that
what babies know is greater, and present much earlier, than once was
suspected. It also established that every baby, right from
birth, is—like a snowflake—different
from every other baby.

JUDITH VIORST

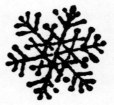

There is nothing more thrilling in this world, I think, than having a child that is yours, and yet is mysteriously a stranger.

AGATHA CHRISTIE

IF THE GREATEST GIFT OF ALL IS LIFE
THEN THE SECOND MUST BE THAT

NO TWO ARE ALIKE.

ANONYMOUS

Your baby is as unique as you are. The chance of another baby having even one fingerprint exactly like your baby's is said to be less than one in sixty-four billion. Even your baby's breathing patterns and sleeping and walking rhythms . . . are as unique as his thumbprint.

EVELYN B. THOMAN, PH.D.

People talk about the miracle of birth. It must be a tremendous experience to see a child being born, your child. Maybe I have no basis for comparison, but the miracle of adoption is an equal miracle. It must be a powerfully exhilarating thing for someone to be able to hand you a living human being. It is the most extraordinary gift you can ever give. There's nothing to match it. And you appreciate having that child so much. That child truly, truly becomes yours. You put your heart on the line for your child.

SUSAN LAUFFERS

Not flesh of my flesh, nor bone of my bone
But still miraculously my own
Never forget for a single moment
You didn't grow under my heart,
But in it.

ANONYMOUS

A close friend called a few days later and asked, "Do you love her yet?" After some time, I answered, "No, I don't think I feel any special attachment to her yet." I agonized over that answer, worrying about what might be wrong with me after all the years of wanting so badly to have a child to love. I cannot tell you exactly when I truly felt love for her. I suspect it developed slowly over the first few weeks. I know that by the time she started smiling at me I felt not only love, but adulation.

CAROLYN JACOBS, ADOPTIVE MOTHER

The ease with which we genuinely love others is directly proportional to our commitment to loving as a priority in our lives. To love is a decision first, an action second, a value next.

KAREN CASEY

Only one person gave me any idea of what having a baby would be like. She said the nearest thing to it was a passionate love affair. I thought she was being silly.

Others had told me, more realistically I thought, of endless diapers, broken nights, runny noses, continual tiredness. I was therefore somewhat dreading the arrival of the baby, whom I was determined not to let disrupt my well-ordered existence.

But as I lay in my hospital bed the day after the birth, everything seemed quite different, and has been ever since. My past life struck me as interesting but rather tawdry, like a bad movie full of stagey love scenes and brittle, competitive people. The reality was here, lying asleep in her cot. . . . I loved her with a love more intense that any I had known before . . .

SALLY EMERSON

In every child who is born, under no matter what circumstances, and of no matter what parents, the potentiality of the human race is born again; and in him, too, once more, and of each of us, our terrific responsibility towards human life; towards the utmost idea of goodness, of the horror of error, and of God.

JAMES AGEE

Within two weeks after your baby is born, you'll realize how selfish you've been all your life. It's an amazing phenomenon.

RUSSELL JOHNSTON

When the nurse took my first child and put him to my breast his tiny mouth opened and reached for me as if he had known forever what to do. He began to suck with such force it took my breath away. It was like being attached to a vacuum cleaner. I began to laugh. I couldn't help myself. It seemed incredible that such a tiny creature could have such force and determination. He too had a purpose. He was raw, insistent and real. With every fibre of his being, this child was drawing his life. And he would not be denied.

Tears of joy ran shamelessly down my cheeks while he sucked. I thought back to my past conviction that only when I had a baby would I know whatever it was I had to know. Now I did know. It is the only important thing I have ever learned, and so ridiculously simple: love exists. It's real and honest and unbelievably solid in a world where far too much is complex or confusing or false.

LESLIE KENTON

But it is an experience of love, and whenever you have an experience of love, it empowers you so much. I feel that I can harness more of myself in life now than I ever could have before.

DIANE CHURCHILL

Love is like a mine. You go deeper and deeper. There are passages, caves, whole strata. You discover entire geological eras.

CHRISTOPHER ISHERWOOD

For love is not like a river, confined between two banks.
Its very essence is to overflow.

MIKE MASON

I'm lying here nursing you, my little boy, and I put in a tape and I just start crying. I'm crying because you're so precious, because I know you won't stay long, and because I don't know why. But I can't stop. This is a different kind of love than I've ever known—I can hardly understand it. It must be from God—maybe something of how He loves us.

JULIE KOVASCKITZ

And every little baby you and I have, or may have, is but another reminder that the most precious Gift heaven ever gave to earth came in the form of a Baby. This was Love personified.

HELEN W. KOOIMAN

We love because He first loved us.

I JOHN 4:19

Natasha's birth transformed my parents in an amazing manner. My father is eighty-two years old and my mother is seventy-six. Both of them, prior to Natasha's birth, carried with them an impending sense of doom. They both realized that they were in the final chapter of their lives and were not enjoying the experience. Natasha has changed their focus. It is quite obvious that they both have a strong desire to live as long as possible so they can enjoy watching their granddaughter grow up. They find every conceivable excuse to drive to our house, which happens to be sixty miles from theirs, just so they can see their granddaughter. They now smile almost as much as our daughter does.

RICHARD L. KATZ

Perfect love sometimes does not come till the first grandchild.

WELSH PROVERB

Life has started all over for me.
The young years of happiness
Have come again in a sweeter form
Than a mother could ever guess.
The love and devotion I gave my child
I thought I could give no other,
But life held a lovely surprise for me—
This year I became a grandmother.

KAY ANDREW

GRANDCHILDREN
ARE THE

CROWN

OF THE AGED.

PROVERBS 17:16

One of the mysteries of life is how the boy who wasn't good enough to marry the daughter can be the father of the smartest grandchild in the world.

ANONYMOUS

There was a tremendous amount of excitement. Finally, at ten that evening the call came. We had a grandson! Oh, I was terribly thrilled!

I flew down to Katherine's the next day. At the hospital they let grandparents in to see the babies. I washed my hands, and put on a white jacket. I went to pick him up, feeling my emotional connection is still with Katherine, for she is my child. But once I held on to that baby, I felt a real connection to him, too. I thought this child is a little bit of me and all those people that made me and went into making Katherine and the same thing from the other side of the family. I was really quite bowled over by it, this sense of connectedness.

PAT MAIN

Grandchildren are the dots that connect the lines from generation to generation.

LOIS WYSE

I suddenly realized that through no act of my own I had become biologically related to a new human being. . . . Somewhere, miles away, a series of events occurred that changed one's own status forever—I had not thought of that and I found it very odd . . .

MARGARET MEAD

When my mother came out to help me during my last week of pregnancy, we hiked, ate out, and fussed over the cats. It was a rare opportunity to spend time alone with her. After the baby was born, she told me she hadn't slept all night and her excitement and automatic love for Mara was very apparent. She was the epitome of the helpful mother during the two weeks following Mara's birth.

I had been such a difficult teenager—I left home when I was nineteen to settle three thousand miles away. Throughout my adulthood, I assumed the residue from that time divided us in subtle ways, but after Mara's birth, I felt a connectedness with my mother when I watched her with my baby. I was amazed to think that she had once treated me exactly the same way. It was beautiful.

NINA FINKEL

For the first time, I could begin to understand a mother's love for her child, and therefore my mother's love for me. As a nonparent, I had heard the words and intellectualized the feelings; but as a mother, I could feel the experience. Now we are both givers of maternal love rather than one a giver and one a recipient. We share this giving and are bound closer together by it. I love this new connection with my mother, and I am grateful that motherhood has enabled me to experience it.

MYRNA FINN

One thing about Sam, one thing about having a baby, is that each step of the way, you simply cannot imagine loving him any more than you already do, because you are bursting with love, loving as much as you are humanly capable of, and then you do; you love him even more.

ANNE LAMOTT

L ove rears the great; love tends the small:
Breaks off the yoke, breaks down the wall:
Accepteth all, fulfilleth all.

Lead lives of love, that others who
Behold your lives may kindle too
With love and cast their lots with you.

HYMN

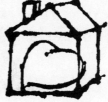

T he most important thing a father can do for his children is to love
their mother.

REV. THEODORE HESBURGH

T his can also be said to wives—making the father secure in their
love is most important in bringing up a happy family. For the
future of the child is dependent upon the continuation and growth
of the love which begot him.

HELEN GOOD BRENNEMAN

THERE ARE ONLY TWO LASTING REQUESTS
WE CAN HOPE TO GIVE
OUR CHILDREN.
ONE OF THESE IS
ROOTS; THE
OTHER, *wings*

HODDING CARTER

What I have learned in the process of raising (four) daughters—
and perhaps it applies to other human affairs as well—is that
there is no single answer, no magic formula, no rigid set of guidelines,
no simple blueprint, no book of easy instructions, no sure way of side-
stepping difficulties, no easy way out. There is love.

GEORGE LEONARD

Before becoming a mother I had a hundred theories on how to bring up children. Now I have seven children and only one theory: love them, especially when they least deserve to be loved.

KATE SAMPERI

Love is always patient and kind. . . . It is always ready to excuse, to trust, to hope, and to endure whatever comes. Love does not come to an end.

I CORINTHIANS 13:4,7-8, *THE JERUSALEM BIBLE*

Love your children with all your hearts, love them enough to discipline them. . . . Praise them for important things, even if you have to stretch them a bit. Praise them a lot. They live on it like bread and butter and they need it more than bread and butter.

LAVINA CHRISTENSEN FUGAL, Mother of the Year, 1955

I am growing my daughter this summer, thrush and all.
Marigolds pale against her golden aura.
Her eyes are snapdragon saucers,
her thighs are dimpled jade plants—rubbery and thick.
She smells of milkwood and daisies.
She clings like a vine but wanders like the Jew.
Her heart-shaped lips are delicate as pussy willow.
Everything about her turns upward—buttercups to light.
This burgeoning bouquet was rooted in my womb.
Next summer I will again plant nasturtium and pansies.
This summer I am growing my daughter, a flower
    extraordinaire.

CAROL KORT

In spite of all the ideas and all the technology and atoms
in the world, it all comes down to shaping one individual at a time.

ANONYMOUS

Our children are not our own. Our children belong to God. He has loaned them to us for a season. . . . They are not ours to keep but to rear. . . . They are not given to us so that we can force them to fulfill our lives and thus, in some way, cancel our failures. They are not tools to be used, but souls to be loved.

THOMAS C. SHORT

Make the most of every day
For time does not stand still.
One day this hand will wave good-bye
While crossing life's brave hill.

ANONYMOUS

There is no end zone. You never cross the goal lines, bite the bullet and do your touchdown dance. I'm 64. Larry, 27.
And he's still my son. He's my son.

PARENTHOOD